Beyond Bedside Manner

Beyond Bedside Manner

Preserving the Vessel For Your Soul's Journey

EVERYTHING YOU NEED TO KNOW TO MAINTAIN
THE SOUL'S CONTAINER THROUGHOUT
THE SECOND HALF OF YOUR LIFE

Jaime G. Corvalan, MD, FACS

Copyright © 2010 by Jaime G. Corvalan, MD, FACS.

Library of Congress Control Number: 2010903315
ISBN: Hardcover 978-1-4500-6001-1
Softcover 978-1-4500-6000-4
Ebook 978-1-4500-6002-8

All rights reserved. No part of this book may be reproduced or transmitted in any form or by any means, electronic or mechanical, including photocopying, recording, or by any information storage and retrieval system, without permission in writing from the copyright owner.

This book was printed in the United States of America.

To order additional copies of this book, contact:
Xlibris Corporation
1-888-795-4274
www.Xlibris.com
Orders@Xlibris.com

CONTENTS

Acknowledgements 9
Introduction: The New Elderhood 11
Chapter One: The New Enlightenment: Defining Age Optimization 17
Chapter Two: Stay in Touch 40
Chapter Three: The Biology of Aging 57
Chapter Four: Food Is A Drug: How To Eat Yourself Young 72
Chapter Five: Nutritional Supplements: What You Need To Know 104
Chapter Six: Going Steady: Hormone Replacement for Men 122
Chapter Seven: You Make Me Feel Like An Optimal Woman: Estrogens, Progesterone, And Testosterone 132
Chapter Eight: A Delicate Balance: Cortisol, Dhea, Melatonin, Thyroid Hormone, and HGH 147
Chapter Nine: The Age Optimization Workout 163
Chapter Ten: Sexual Healing: Tapping Into the Real Fountain of Youth 176

Epilogue: Just the Beginning 185
Resources: Lab Testing 191
Glycemic Food Index Guide 195
References 199
Index 221

DEDICATION

For my father, who told me when I was a child: "Nothing can bring you down, son, unless you let it." His words and his example became ingrained in my being and have allowed me to both reach great heights and to rebound after great falls, including his own passing. Because of the character, integrity, and honor of my father, I can face the unknown future with clarity and mind and peace in my heart.

And I dedicate this book to my mother, who I lost to death when I was only nine. She left with me an indelible imprint of gentleness and soft, loving kindness. Her nurturing spirit remains a vital force within my own soul. In the short time I was privileged to love and be loved by her, she bestowed upon me the gift of empathy and abiding love that I have been fortunate enough to share with my family, friends and patients. Thank you, Mother, for teaching me to love and honor myself and to look for the best in all people.

ACKNOWLEDGEMENTS

I WOULD LIKE TO give special recognition to Melissa Lynn Block for her patient collaboration and skills in concretizing my ideas from concept to form. She is an editor whose ability to weave together the complexities of science and the depths of the humanities which has been of great value to me. Thank you also to my loving wife, Christine; my good friend Mike Chupa, who was a valuable sounding board for many of the ideas that ended up in these pages; my son Brent, an amazing young man who possesses wisdom well beyond his years; Cenegenics, for giving me the idea to write this book and for teaching me a great deal about optimal health; the patients who entrust their health to me; and the office staff that has given me indispensable support as I have juggled writing, doctoring, family life and learning over the past five years.

INTRODUCTION

The New Elderhood

HUMAN BEINGS, FOR the first time in recorded history, have a very good chance of living into a second century. Think about it. If you're fifty, you could have forty or even fifty years or more to live.

Have you considered how you intend to live all those extra years?

You have a great many choices—far more than any group of human beings has had in the history of our species. Even a century ago, it was a big deal to live into old age at all, and there were no opportunities to spend one's golden years watching television, going on cruises, moving to a senior citizens' community in Florida or Arizona, eating at all-you-can-eat buffets, or planning trips to see your grandchildren in faraway places. These kinds of choices are new to us human beings. Such abundance of choice is a wonderful thing, as are many extra decades of health in which to indulge in it.

These considerations are every bit as important as any about outliving your savings—which the AARP tells us is more likely than ever to happen. You might only be halfway through with your years on earth. You do have a second chance.

As a physician who specializes in Age Optimization—where we use medical and nutritional therapies to create optimal health and well-being at every age—I've assembled all you need to know to take the best possible care of yourself after the age of forty. This book offers a thorough introduction to all the elements of a comprehensive self-care program for people who are looking into their second six decades with hope and excitement. It addresses mostly physical concerns; but as physical and psychological/emotional concerns are inextricably intertwined, there are also chapters designed to help with mental and emotional obstacles to total health, as well as those that arise from dysfunctional relationships.

This is not a book about trying to live forever, or even about trying to live past the natural lifespan of human beings through any artificial means. Let's acknowledge that constant awareness of death is an absolute necessity for a life well lived. As we grow comfortable with the constant presence of our own mortality, consciousness is quickened. It becomes easy to differentiate the trivial from the enduring and meaningful. And we can tune into that which lives beneath the eternal flux, the cycling of death and life. Our physical life is the blossom, which passes; the soul remains forever, re-integrating into the eternal when the body passes on.

Death is not something to be avoided or feared. It's the freeing of the soul from the bounds of matter, and the return of that soul to the oneness of the spirit realm. This book is about preserving that vessel in as energized and healthy a state as possible so that we can have plenty of time for—and minimal distractions from—entering into our true life's journey. How we approach the meaning of this journey is closely tied to our mindfulness that it will end.

Until its re-incorporation into the Great Spirit, the soul needs a physical body in which to live out its adventure and to reinforce its purpose in this life. In this vessel, the soul lives out its particular myth, going through many metamorphoses, stages, and rites of passage. The soul needs the body in order to have its human experience. The body is a temporary vessel that is animated by the soul; the soul comes from a transcendent realm with a specific purpose and meaning. If the word 'soul' makes you uncomfortable, replace it with the word 'psyche,' or vital energy, or prana, or chi—whatever you want to call that which enters the body when life begins and leaves it when life ends.

The soul needs time and the right environment for the unfolding of its meaning and unlimited knowledge within each individual vessel—time and safety to do, unfold, create, and manifest. And today, we are finding that we have more time to refine and polish this expression. The purpose of any Age Optimization program, then, is not simply to preserve the vessel so that it looks nice and is fun to play around in and dress up—it's to actively participate in the blessing of an increased life span by moving towards more evolved levels of consciousness.

People have treated their bodies without reverence, allowing them to become polluted with toxins, poisons of all kinds, oxidative stress radicals, fats, and inflammation. We have run them day in and out until absolute exhaustion, worked like workaholics. In that process our bodies have been disowned. We have divorced ourselves from much of the substance that makes us human.

To become remarried to the body means to maintain it in a fit, active, ready, and energized state. This, in turn, requires that you learn to manage and optimally adapt to stress, optimize diet and nutritional supplements, regularly exercise at an intensity adequate for physical fitness, and (possibly) use bio-identical hormone therapy—topics covered in depth in these pages. This comprehensive approach can provide you with the ideal vessel for living an optimal life throughout your years, but particularly after middle age. The aim of Age Optimization is to maintain the body at a level of function achievable in one's forties.

This having been said, be warned that this is not an "anti-aging" book. Although it will give you detailed information about how to eat, drink, exercise, relate, and use nutritional supplements, it does not give hard and fast formulas. As much as it is about tools for maintaining your health, it is about finding meaning and purpose in your life, particularly in the second half of life—a sort of *proactive* aging. But in the end, no matter what ends you go to in your efforts to preserve your body, optimizing your life during these years is an inside job.

Any person who wants to optimize his age will need to do some serious preventive and maintenance work on his body and soul. This book will be your guide. We explore every possible avenue for the preservation of physical health. The goal is to provide each person with a seaworthy, efficient vessel into which to sail through what can be the most productive and satisfying years of one's life.

Today's health care debate accepts, at its foundation, that millions of people are going to be sick and will need drugs and surgery and nursing home care, and asks how we're going to pay for all these surgical, medical, and pharmacological interventions; extravagantly costly medical equipment, auxiliary support; and accompanying emotional, physical, and spiritual suffering from alienation, loneliness, and abandonment. I propose, instead, that we base this debate on the presupposition that we can make people way more alert, more deliberate, and more proactive about their health. When? Before physical decline begins—believe it or not, at about age thirty. With wholehearted disease prevention and Age Optimization beginning before middle age, it is possible to keep most people healthy enough so that they don't need hospitalization or pharmaceuticals or become drug addicts for life. Even if you are already well into middle age, there is much you can do to preserve your vessel.

Most Americans over fifty take one or several prescription drugs every day, indefinitely, and think nothing of it. We are a culture that thinks it can solve just about any problem with pharmaceuticals. Pharmaceutical companies have been allowed to use sophisticated advertisements to convert individuals into pharmaceutical consumers. Our government protects the interests of these companies, and the medical organizations have played right into this by enabling it. They tell young people to "just say no" to drugs and sex while advertising better living through pharmaceutical chemistry on TV, radio, and in newspapers, and with a pervasive message that popping a pill for any perceived discomfort or minor pain is something we can just do. We are so brainwashed that we think this is not only OK but that it is safe and necessary.

Old-guard medicine's consciousness is about power and not about healing; it talks about killing the disease with magic bullets before it can kill us. It is a war mentality. The consciousness of the new medicine is love, care, protection, prevention, and cultivation of healing. The new medicine is about

- honoring nature and allowing it to help reestablish and maintain the homeostasis of the body's own healing capacity;
- learning to manage stress and create a positive adaptation to this inescapable entity;
- how we think, feel, and create nurturing relationships, understanding clearly the vital role they play in keeping us content and well;

- keeping away from those relationships (to people, jobs, stressors, foods) that are the opposite of nurturing—those that are making us ill.

The purpose of this book is to help you have the best possible life, which in turn will enable you to contribute in making a better world for yourself and for all. You will need a healthy body to do this. To have a healthy body, certain steps must be taken—steps that include giving up certain ways of eating and living and shifting to new ways. This is easier said than done and may require some shifts in consciousness, thinking, and attitudes. This book is also designed to help you with that. To make a better world for all, we need to allow, empower, and motivate our own greatness without making it a source of personal pride. This greatness does not serve just the ego. It can (and should) be channeled through a healthy body and out into the world.

When people talk about getting healthy or losing weight, it is usually for the purpose of improving one's appearance and having more power in attracting other people's attentions. This doesn't last. With Age Optimization, you stand a good chance of having enough time to find the heaven on earth where you can transcend all lack and selfishness. Stunningly rapid evolution in nature and science is providing us with resources that can keep us strong and youthful even as we live longer. But all this is of little use if we don't acknowledge that we, as a species, are at a turning point in our evolution of consciousness and that living long and healthy is about more than selfish ego concerns.

To reach the part of you that is not the ego—the part that wants redemption, where our opposites can be held together, becoming one at the center, whole, and complete—requires significant chronological time. Yet the choices being made by most people today are not buying time in a healthy body. They are destructive and deadly. Making healthier choices will drastically raise the odds of maintaining health, energy, and even sexual passion and enjoyment throughout the second half of your life.

To make healthier choices, you will need to become *health literate*. Real health literacy will give you the motivation to stick with healthful choices for life. Reading this book will make you health literate. It's health literacy, not any simple, quick "Band-aid" diet or fitness fad, that will optimize your chances of living a healthy, long, energetic life. Health literacy doesn't stand alone, however. It is not just *information*; it's the awakening of *awareness*. No matter what prescription you are offered, if you do not take the time to become aware and present to your feelings and your experience, I guarantee you will end up right back where you started.

Just between you and I, we can't count on young people to handle the world's problems. They have energy and passion, but they don't have the strength and maturity to bring solutions full circle. It's not time for you to step off the scene yet. You are still very much needed in the world. The evolution of this planet is counting on your awareness.

Get ready; it's time to optimize yourself.

CHAPTER ONE

The New Enlightenment: Defining Age Optimization

We must take responsibility for the way we feel. The notion that others can make us feel good or bad is untrue. Consciously or—more frequently—unconsciously, we are choosing how we feel at every single moment. The external world is in so many ways a mirror of our beliefs and expectations. Why we feel the way we feel is the result of the symphony and harmony of our own molecules of emotion that affect every aspect of our physiology, producing blissful good health or miserable disease.

—Candace Pert, *Molecules of Emotion*

A FEW YEARS ago, I heard a story about a group of people trapped in a mineshaft. They were completely cut off from outside air and knew they would all perish for lack of oxygen if they were not rescued soon.

A couple of the men who were wearing watches volunteered to keep track of the time so that all could know how long they had been trapped. Being good Samaritans, the timekeepers conspired to divide the number of hours by two: For every two days they were underground, they told the others that only a single day had gone by.

The group was actually rescued in about fourteen days. All but those with the watches believed that only seven days had elapsed. Everyone but the timekeepers survived.

Finding the "fountain of youth" starts with recognizing that time is a human construct. It does not exist anywhere but in the human consciousness. Consciousness is the way we interpret—and make—reality in our minds.

Awareness, on the other hand, is immediate experience, without interpretation. Those trapped people died because they absolutely *knew* they should be and, no doubt, *were* out of oxygen. This was their consciousness of their situation. This was the story they told themselves, and it had enough power over their bodies to end their lives. The others were simply aware and present, and they still had oxygen to breathe, and they survived.

Our conceptions of time and aging have similarly huge effects on our physical well-being. We can shift those conceptions. Carlos Castaneda said that life is a feeling after a feeling after a feeling. It is not what you think or what you do, or what timeline you are on or think you're on. Your life is composed of what you feel from moment to moment.

The ancient Greeks had two versions of time: *chronos* time and *kayros* time. Chronos time was the sequence of days, years, months; kayros time was eternal time: moment after moment after moment. Kayros time is the continually flowing present, the *now*. We can choose to exist in kayros time.

This having been said, the fact is, your body changes as you grow older. There is a lot you can do about the less pleasant aspects of those changes. You can do a lot to prevent so-called diseases of aging like heart disease, cancer, dementia, and diabetes—all of which are widely held to be inevitable aspects of aging.

HEALTH LITERACY BASICS

Virtually all medical minds agree that to slow the aging process, you should eat moderately, avoid processed foods and excessive sun exposure, maintain a healthful weight, exercise, and do what you can to minimize the impact of stress. Some recommend nutritional supplements and hormones; some merely recommend them as adjuncts to a healthful diet and exercise while others seem to believe that hormones or supplements are a sort of fountain of youth.

A huge number of fad diets and workout programs have sprung from the basic tenets of healthful living. We hear these programs described as "groundbreaking" or "revolutionary" or that its creator will share the earth-shattering "secrets" for a model-trim, wrinkle-free body and total well-being. Most of these fad programs claim that specific, small alterations in diet or activity will overhaul your health. But anyone who has tried one or more of these programs knows that they don't work. This hasn't stopped Americans from spending about $35 billion per year on weight loss and diet products.

What does work? Foundational change in your level of moment-to-moment awareness: your level of presence in this very moment. This is the only thing that breaks you free from habitual behaviors that cause you to eat unhealthfully and otherwise take poor care of the only body you will ever have, the greatest gift you've ever received. Ninety-five percent of those who try to change their eating habits or lifestyles might see success for a while but eventually backslide, and this happens *because they remain unaware and health-illiterate.*

The first step toward the kind of awareness that will optimize your health is what I call *health literacy*. A health-literate person knows how his body works and what effect food, stress, and physical activity have on that body. Once you become health literate, you will dismiss fads and diet plans out of hand because you will know how to make good choices without any prescription from a fitness trainer or diet guru trying to make a few bucks off your health illiteracy.

Health literacy means having a basic understanding of

- food and how it affects your body and mind;
- how to eat to optimize health, reduce risk of most diseases, and create abundant energy.

The understanding of these first two points, combined, adds up to what I call *food literacy*. Add to this an understanding of

- how your thoughts and level of awareness affect your physical health and how you can shape those thoughts in health-promoting ways;

- how to wisely, safely use the nutritional supplements that have real support in the scientific literature;
- how stress kills and what to do about it;
- how the natural decline of certain hormones ages you, and what to do about it—and you have the foundations of health literacy and of Age Optimization.

We know which behaviors lead us down the road to age-related diseases: sugary desserts, breads, rice and potatoes, marbled meat, and sedentary hours in front of the TV or computer. We know those same behaviors make us fat and tired. We don't need expensive Hollywood nutritional consultants to tell us this stuff—it's rudimentary.

What most diets and health fads fail to address is this: *What truly motivates us to make healthful changes?* The gorgeous celebrity trainer who pushes you to eat this way or the handsome diet expert who promotes the latest fad diet that does not inspire awareness? They only give information. This is why over 90 percent of people who lose weight regain it within five years.

Consider the word *diet* itself. This word was initially a medical term. A sick person in the hospital might have to go on a soft diet, a liquid diet, a bland diet, or an NPO (nothing *per os,* or nothing by mouth) diet. When she gets better, she goes off the diet. Diets are, by nature, restrictive. Diets are for sick people!

Perhaps this word *diet* needs to be struck from our vocabulary. I use it in this book because it's the commonly accepted word for the foods people eat, but I do so begrudgingly. Diets are insulting. Do you need so-called authorities telling you, "You're too stupid to know what to eat, so we'll tell you"? You *do* know what to eat to be healthy. I promise you! Do you really think that you're eating healthy food when you consume that greasy bag of fast-food french fries and soda? Is there any doubt in your mind or your body when you've consumed a meal that enhances your health—"Oh, maybe I shouldn't have eaten all that salad and brown rice and poached wild-caught salmon"?

What you need to know is *how foods interact in and with your body* and *how combinations of foods work in your body.* This is food literacy, and once you possess it, you will no sooner make french fries a staple of your diet as you would drive 100 mph on a motorcycle without a helmet.

Right now, you may not truly comprehend how damaging junk food is to your body or how healing and beneficial the good food choices are. This will change as you read this book and become food literate. Your problem in that moment of french fry madness is that you are not *aware* of how those greasy morsels are aging and destroying you one bite at a time. Even if you know in some part of your brain that you shouldn't eat them, you have an ability to allow, or ignore, its cries to be drowned out by the momentary bliss of stuffing your mouth with crispy, salty, fatty morsels of potato. Food literacy will give you the knowledge you need to be present and aware of when it's time to eat. You'll be one of those people who others look at as having amazing willpower, saying "no thanks" to all the foods they can't resist!

If we know, deeply, what the wrong foods are doing to our bodies and how the right foods honor and strengthen our bodies, we can stay in awareness and make the right choice every time.

Now this does not mean that you won't have sacrifices to make. Nothing good happens in this world without sacrifice.

ON SACRIFICE

Most people think that sacrifice means giving something up, or forgoing what you want. But the origin of the word sacrifice means something quite different: it means *to make sacred* or *make holy*. Sacrifice is the art of drawing energy from one level and reinvesting it in another to produce a higher form of consciousness. Sacrifice is never life denying; rather, it is life affirming.

Sacrifice is not giving up something to get something else you want more. It is not giving up cookies on one day so that you may eat cake the next. It is an interior event. A sacrifice made for the sake of thinner thighs or some other person's happiness is depleting, but sacrifice is always life affirming when offered to a transpersonal self greater than you—you may call it God, or a Higher Power. When you let go of an unhealthy want, you are not giving something up as much as you are surrendering to the flow of what is best for you and everyone in the world. Ultimately, sacrifice is about making a different conscious choice than what you have made until today. Sacrifice is also about humility, gratitude, and willingness to give back to the world.

WHAT IS AGE OPTIMIZATION?

You have a new chance, a second opportunity to live a long life in a body that's in great working order. This is, most fundamentally, what Age Optimization is about: taking advantage of advances in science and medicine, depth psychology and physical training to achieve a body that's strong, healthy, and pleasant for you to live in and enjoy, with a mind that is alert, clear, content, defenseless, and capable of authentic love and gratitude without regrets. It is about always looking into how to reach that which is optimum in every aspect of life and living—physically, spiritually, mentally, and emotionally.

Age Optimization is a comprehensive program designed to anticipate and minimize the chances of health problems that require medical or surgical intervention in the aging process, allowing us to spend the second half of our lives in a healthy, energized, active, and emotionally fulfilled state. This journey may involve losing weight, managing stress, raising awareness, improving relationships, or some combination of these. It draws from current research in the fields of aging, nutrition, medicine, depth psychology, and spirituality to redefine being fifty, sixty, seventy, eighty, ninety, or one hundred years old and beyond—making aging something quite different from what it was in our parents' day.

Age Optimization does not involve suppressing symptoms of disease. Symptoms are not diseases; they are messages from deep within the body that something is out of balance. We need to learn how to translate that message and act on it. Today, millions of "seniors" take multiple prescription drugs to control symptoms such as arthritis and high blood pressure, to prevent decreased insulin sensitivity (which can lead to type 2 diabetes) or high cholesterol. These conditions are *symptoms of imbalance*, not true diseases. While controlling such symptoms with medications may help prevent serious issues like heart attack, so much more can be done to rebalance the body and eliminate the need for most or all these medications. If we remedy the source of the imbalance, the problem is solved, and symptoms go away on their own.

Age Optimization seeks to eliminate symptoms at their root, using whatever is known that works. That might, in the end, involve one or more drugs (for example, statins or Viagra), dietary changes, nutritional supplements, hormones, surgery, exercises, psychoanalysis, psychological counseling, or spiritual searching. This is not "alternative medicine" or "natural medicine"—it's a meeting of the most advanced modern medical science with the long-effective tradition of natural healing.

Instead of waging a destructive and futile war to kill terrorists one at a time, we should find out what is creating the terrorists in the first place and deal with the source. The same goes for the "terrorists" in your body!

WINNING THE WAR ON FAT

When people are illiterate, they are easily duped and exploited. America is a nation of food illiterates. Remember how Bill Clinton used to go jogging, but he also famously loved fast food? He ended up with five-vessel disease and had to have bypass surgery before he turned sixty. Without that, he would have died—indeed, he could have dropped dead at any minute before that surgery. He became food literate and aware. Now he's raising billions to help with health care and other causes around the world.

A fat person is not a well person. The more excess fat you carry around, the more your body is producing inflammatory chemicals. The truth is, people who really do eat well *consistently*, making the best possible choices over months, years, and decades, have a difficult time becoming and staying fat. This consistency is what Age Optimization is all about.

Overweight and obese individuals are at increased risk for many diseases and health conditions, including the following:

- Hypertension (high blood pressure)
- Osteoarthritis (a degeneration of cartilage and its underlying bone within a joint)

- Dyslipidemia (for example, high total cholesterol or high levels of triglycerides)
- Type 2 diabetes
- Coronary heart disease
- Stroke
- Gallbladder disease
- Sleep apnea and respiratory problems
- Some cancers (endometrial, breast, prostate, and colon)
- Dementia

One doesn't very often see a person who is both obese and elderly. This is why.

In 2007, health care spending in the United States was over $2.2 trillion dollars—just under $7,500 per U.S. resident, or 16.2 percent of expenditures for goods and services. This represented the largest one-year increase in health care spending in the history of the nation. Over the eleven years that passed between 1995 and 2006, health care spending increased by 64 percent. This is partly due to the aging of the American population and to more aggressive, early treatment of illnesses that once were not detected until much later in their progression; but obesity, poor eating habits in the population, and poor self-care play a significant role as well. As of 2002, an estimated 11.6 percent of health care expenses were related to obesity and excessive weight. Sixty percent of medical costs in the United States are associated with chronic conditions, which are often associated with poor nutrition and lack of physical activity. According to research published in the *Journal of the American Medical Association* (*JAMA*), poor nutrition and lack of physical activity are responsible for three hundred thousand to six hundred thousand preventable deaths each year.[1]

THE ROLE OF AWARENESS

So many patients come to me with bodies that are broken, and they want me to fix the broken parts. They have prediabetes, a lot of fat in the

---

[1] McGinnis JM, Foege WH, "Actual causes of death in the United States," *JAMA* 1993 Nov 10; 270 (18): 2207-12.

omentum (the viscera, the area within the abdomen beneath the abdominal muscle wall) and on their frames as well as a host of other problems. Their worst problem is that they don't want to change. They think that they can't change. They believe that they are powerless to change.

Optimizing one's age is fundamentally not only about looking better (although it will help you to do that too). It's about keeping our bodies and souls in optimal condition so that we can take advantage of the wisdom that comes with getting older and find meaning in our lives. We can find new levels of peace, happiness, and sensual joy. We can feel good in our bodies.

Like any physician who cares about making people well (as opposed to just temporarily fixing their broken parts and sending them on their way), I have my own guidelines about how to eat, how to live, and what supplements to take. Although these guidelines can be specific and detailed, they are all strongly supported by scientific research; and for years I have seen their positive, life-changing results, with both myself and hundreds of my patients.

But before I share that information with you, let's lay the foundation of this plan—what is often the crucial, missing ingredient: lasting, powerful awareness and reverence for life, with soulful self-motivation.

The human being who gorges himself ever day on junk food, or doesn't get any exercise, or performs work that he doesn't believe in, or engages in unhealthy interpersonal relationships, is not living in an aware state. And until the person is ready to embrace awareness, he cannot make the best choices.

Awareness is the lifeline that connects us to the seat of the soul, a sacred place where our inner world meets the outer. It is also the seat of our *feeling* selves.

It is not about *understanding* or *thinking about* or *analyzing* what we experience; that goes on in the abstraction of the mind. Awareness is about *observing without judgment* and being here, in this moment, with *what is,* right now.

The moment we pass judgment, the minute we formulate an opinion or think about the past or the future, we thrust ourselves out of awareness and the experience of simply observing and knowing.

Here are some exercises to help you become more aware:

- Throughout the day, pause to become aware of *this very moment*. Look, observe, listen, and breathe.
- Listen to the chatter of your thoughts. Please know that this chatter is not you; it is made up of dark voices from the past that create neurotic fear in your mind. This chatter is an excellent reflection of your beliefs—those that serve you and those that don't. If you're like most people, your self-talk jumps all over the place and is by turns overly critical or overconfident, and it wallows regularly in negativity. No one can change their self-talk right away. Just begin by listening to it. Imagine that it is not you but the voices of strangers from your past. They are a reflection of your beliefs. As you recognize beliefs that don't serve you now, you can gently guide this internal chatter into a more constructive language . . . more on this in a bit.
- When you have strong negative emotions, simply acknowledge them and allow them to move through you, without blame or doubt. Suppressing feelings you don't like becomes a source of great unresolved stress that will make you old in body and lacking in spiritual vitality. You don't have to *do* anything about them because they are not you; they are only responses to memories and old thoughts. And they are here now to teach you something about you and are no one else's responsibility.
- See and experience the actual person with whom you are interacting. Don't compare that person to any other, but observe him or her as a unique individual. Look carefully at and relate to what you experience with this person and not those beliefs, misconceptions, or fantasies that you might have about him or her. Similarly, when someone is trying to relate to *you*, stop and listen as though your life depended on it.
- Remind yourself often to use your senses (seeing, hearing, touching, smelling, tasting). Breathe in the smells, look at what's around you—whether you're pushing a cart through Wal-Mart or frolicking in a green forest. Sense your own body in three-dimensional space, letting go of time.
- With no distractions, experience your meals as you are eating them. Enjoy your food slowly and completely. Be grateful for it. Taste thoroughly: you might find that although you thought you

loved fried chicken, if you pay close attention while eating it, it's not nearly as wonderful as you thought. In the hours following a meal, keep a close watch on how you are feeling. How do you feel after eating a bag of greasy chips versus a lush green salad? How do you feel two hours after a gooey piece of cake? Notice. Pay attention. Let those sensations of discomfort and fatigue inform your next choice.

THE ROLE OF BELIEF

Beliefs are shortcuts we all take. They save us the time required to think something through. If we know what we believe, we can shoot out a quick answer or make a snap decision. But this cancels out awareness. Some beliefs become fundamental to our personalities, allowing us to make quick judgments and decisions in our day-to-day lives.

When I advise my patients on how to eat, use replacement hormones, exercise, and take nutritional supplements, I do so in the fervent hope that they will use their extended years and energy to live contented, soulful, purposeful lives, and that a new consciousness will evolve into a higher level of awareness. Most often, to do this, they need to question their current beliefs.

What is a belief? It is an idea, a thought, which has been solidified and will not change without being questioned in an intensive, direct way. Your thoughts, your awareness, and your choices are channeled through these solid points; or more accurately, your thoughts, awareness, and choices smash into your beliefs and are irrevocably changed in the process. *In order to change your behavior, you will need to recognize and question your beliefs.*

You can do this. Your beliefs are based on little more than your upbringing and your past experiences; and you can program new, better, supportive beliefs into the present moment. Beliefs can become channels for beneficial awareness. They can lead you to make great choices without even thinking about it.

If you believe that you cannot live without daily pizza, chocolate bars, and double espressos, that belief has to change. If you believe that you are not on this planet to do something marvelous, that belief has to change. Otherwise, you're fighting a battle of wills that you are going to lose. Your beliefs will undermine even your most dramatic display of willpower.

As you work with your system of beliefs, remember that beliefs are not right or wrong. We usually do not even know they are there, but once we become aware of them, we can change them simply by questioning their validity. They're only tools, not truths.

How do you change a belief? By asking yourself better questions. When you bump up against a belief, question it. As soon as you ask a better question, you immediately change the focus, the meaning, which will, in turn, immediately affect the outcome.

We need to question in a specific way. Certainly you've heard the biblical aphorism, "Ask and you shall receive." To that I add my own: "Ask poor questions and you'll get poor results." If you ask stupid questions like "Why does this always happen to me?" you'll stay shallow and receive stupid answers that will not move you to a newer and better place.

If you ask disempowering questions, you are disempowering your responses and yourself. To become a more powerful pilot of your own life, ask better questions and let the answers come with fascination, curiosity, and wonder—the keys to being successful and optimized, healthy and younger!

A friend sent me an e-mail that read:

> *I think maybe you can help me with the issue of empowering/disempowering questions when it comes to financial matters. I am terrible at managing my money and have a hard time even imagining making it grow. I desperately want to own a home and save for retirement and pay off my credit cards. My business is taking off and yet I still never have anything to show for it . . . I am broke, and deep in debt, always behind, always stressed about money. I'm sick of it. How do I change this?*

Let's look at the language: "*Terrible* at managing his money." He has a *hard time* imagining himself wealthy. He is *desperate* to own a home, save for retirement, and pay off debts. He's *sick* of this problem. These words all reflect an image of self as a failure. Deep in our psyche, time stands still. For this person, some early loss created a shock in his psyche and is still reverberating. This will manifest in an irrational fear, such as the fear of failure or powerlessness. These fears translate to being incapable of losing weight or optimizing the body.

What we are facing in a situation like this is something from our childhood that we placed in old memory "folders" with names like I Can't, I Will Never Be Able To, I Will Never Get Better, or I Will Fall Apart. We remain held trapped in the past. The more you remain in your mind, the less you will be in touch with your body. This is neurotic fear: the inability to handle what we feel or how powerless we may be. This is not fearing the thing itself but our powerlessness in the face of it. We come to believe that we are defenseless and resourceless.

Neurotic fear hides its real face and goes by many aliases: worry, inhibition, inability, indecision, reluctance, embarrassment. They all mean "I am scared." Neurotic fears believe that things will never change. This is illusory because nothing stays the same all the time. I asked my friend with the financial troubles to get into a high state of joy—to remember, in a visceral way, a time when he had such joy. I told him that the essence of joy is empowerment. That it recharges your lively energies. Once you have that feeling of joy, you can then say with energy, "I can and I will and I trust that I can handle whatever comes up!"

I suggested that he begin to ask *positive* questions and make positive statements: "How can I learn to manage my money better?" or "How can I learn to become wealthy?"

Talk and think about what you *do* want, not what you don't want. Create an image in your mind of what you want and let it be real to you that it will happen. *See yourself getting what you want.* Let your attitudes and beliefs go in the direction of you having what you want. Don't look for someone else to give it to you—not any diet plan, workout fad, or clinic. It's all on you: all the awareness that there is no wealth without giving, and all the joy in accomplishing what you set out to do.

Think of the example of billionaire Andrew Carnegie, who wrote down a plan when a young man and left it in his safe. It said, simply, "In the first half of my life, I plan to make a large fortune; and in the second half of my life, I plan to give it all away to charities." Today, it's hard to look at the donors to any big charitable organization without seeing the Carnegie Foundation on the list.

Thinking and talking positively works for your health too. Want to be thinner? Don't say, "I just can't seem to lose this weight!" or ask, "Why can't I lose this weight?" Avoid blaming statements like "I hate how I look," "It's Mom's fault for feeding me all those french fries when I was a kid!" or "Everyone in my family is this way." Ask yourself a powerful new question, such as "How can I change my eating and exercise patterns so that I can be a size four again?" and you will receive the answers, in *becoming aware that you can obtain anything that you really want if you believe that you can.*

Look ahead. Ask *possibility* questions, not disempowering questions. Make positive statements. "I'm going to feel so great when I'm thinner. I'm going to hike up mountains and walk on the beach in my bathing suit!" "I will live a long, healthy, youthful, and happy life."

Don't see problems; see *situations*. Ask what's great about your situation right now. What is it teaching you? And what can you do with all the tools at your disposal? The manner in which you deal with setbacks, disappointments, and frustrations will shape your life more than anything else.

Be specific about what you want. Instead of saying, "I just want to lose some weight," which is a statement of preference, say, "I will lose fifteen pounds before June 1." This prepares you to succeed, as long as you give yourself enough time. (Asking to lose more than five to eight pounds a month could prove difficult for most people and set you up to gain all the weight back and then some).

Once you decide what you want, *specifically,* ask yourself good questions about how to take action. Notice whether your approach is working or not. And be flexible, changing what you are doing as many times as necessary until you get the results you want.

Listen to and question your self-talk. If you just listen, you will notice that this talk is the same as it was yesterday, a month ago, a year ago . . . and these are your beliefs, and they are stopping you.

Beliefs are the map, and the map is not the territory. The description is not the described. What are you telling yourself? Realize that people have between sixty thousand and seventy thousand thoughts *every day*, and they are usually the same day after day after day after day. How are you describing your world? What you are supposed to be and have? Thinking differently will make a huge difference. Instead of "I'm too fat, I wish I was healthier, I wish I could be more athletic, I wish I didn't have to worry about croaking from a heart attack like my father did," see yourself as those things and state clearly, "I want to and I will be healthy, slender, athletic, I will take excellent care of my heart."

You create your reality. Why not create a reality that is optimized? Tell yourself this, from *A Course in Miracles*: "I am responsible for what I see. I choose the feelings I experience and I decide upon the goal I wish to achieve. And everything that happens to me I ask for and receive as I have asked."

When negative self-talk comes up, simply listen to it, acknowledge it, learn from it, and release it. You can visualize a balloon floating away or a rock you've tossed off a cliff and into the ocean or a leaf being carried downstream. Let go of judgments, the dwelling on old insults and injuries, and the obsessing about the future. It's all just noise that clutters your mind.

You don't have to analyze or resolve it. Send it out into the universe with love! Say, "Thank you! Now I can let you go."

Then take action and be flexible. Keep moving forward.

TELL YOURSELF: I CANNOT FAIL!

Nobody can fail without his or her own permission. Failure is a judgment. Therefore you can choose success. You can choose to never fail. You can choose to be a winner.

Fear will either paralyze you or motivate you to take action. It's energy. Use it. Anytime you feel intimidated or nervous about something, go to a private place and jump up and down. Hit the bed with a pillow. Jump for a minute or so or hit a post with a wet towel and yell, "I am unstoppable,

unstoppable, unstoppable, unstoppable!" Think, "I cannot fail!" Go ahead, yell it out loud, many times over. Yell out the thing that you *want to believe* to get you to where you want to go.

I often remind myself that I am unstoppable, that I cannot fail or, more accurately, that every so-called failure is simply a mistake that taught me something of value. I can then ask myself, "What could I have done differently?" There is no learning without making mistakes. No remorse, only resiliency. You cannot learn to succeed without making mistakes! But you also cannot let yourself perceive mistakes as failures because this will stop you in your tracks.

Seen from this perspective, mistakes are learning tools. When you pair this positive outlook with the right knowledge—the knowledge of how your body works and what you can do to promote its health—you're on your way to optimization.

THE IMPORTANCE OF THE FEELING FUNCTION

In most modern Western cultures, people are afraid of their feelings. So afraid, in fact, and from such an early age, that we begin to do all we can to avoid feeling much of anything. By adulthood, many of us find ourselves unable to identify our feelings at all. We rationalize this by saying that feelings aren't worth paying attention to, anyhow, as they are not to be trusted. We put our faith in reason, logic, and thought instead.

But in 1921, Carl Jung made a revolutionary statement that is as true today as it was then: that *feeling*, as a function of consciousness, is equal to thinking, sensing, and intuiting. This insight has held through modern times. We cannot have conscious comprehension without feeling and thinking because both are rational functions. Feelings appreciate and relate; they are instrumental for attributing value and making judgments. Feelings give hope, stir longings, and give direction to one's life.

How do you know what you want in your heart of hearts? Your feelings will tell you, if you listen. Feelings assign value to life's experiences; they are rational, but do not follow logic, which is mental and abstract. Our feelings move us to experience life in real time and motivate us to move toward what we perceive as good or pleasurable and away from that which we perceive as painful or dangerous. It is our feelings that give value to our experiences.

Feelings do more than show us the way to what we truly want or keep us from that which we don't want. How they are felt or not felt has an enormous impact on the aging process and upon our relationships. A healthy way of acknowledging and coping with feelings is an indispensable tool in defusing the deadly effects of stress, a topic I'll address in more detail throughout the remainder of this book. Unless you get in touch with how you feel, you remain in a reactive mode, doing things that hurt your body, life, and relationships.

Emotion describes the changing physiological state of the body in response to changes in feeling and thinking states. Emotion is not the same as feeling. Emotion is an affect that follows a thought. When you feel fear and get butterflies in the stomach and on the back of your neck the hairs stand up, or you feel sadness and then you cry, it is because you are having an emotional response that you don't like. Emotions quite often appear removed from the present moment; for example, you have an emotional response when you remember an event that triggered powerful feelings of loss in you.

Stop for a moment and get in touch with how you are feeling, right now. Do so not by searching for words to describe your feelings or by thinking about how you *should* be feeling. Just identify the sensations in your chest, your muscles, and your gut. Once you do this, you will know what you feel. You don't have to even put words to it. Just be there for a moment.

Were your feelings at this moment a surprise to you? Have you been denying these feelings, and if so, for how long? How long have you been ignoring them, invalidating them, or waiting for them to just go away? Did they threaten to overwhelm you?

In our culture, there is so little time for feelings and for getting in touch with them because feelings are uncomfortable. Instead of being, we tend to prefer doing, which is about thinking: mental and abstract. Bad feelings are labeled with terms like *depression* or *anxiety*. Even when they're medicated with antidepressants or other drugs, these feelings live on, beneath our radar, instead of being brought out into the open and moved through. And no wonder, if we allow these feelings to come to the surface, we may be forced to recognize that we have to make some big changes in our lives.

The truth is, however, that we can't afford to *not* get in touch with our feelings. Suppressed feelings stew inside us, causing ill health, discord, and disruption in our lives and relationships. Our feelings represent one of the highest forms of knowing, helping us to know how much value to place in an experience. They speak straight from the soul. Listening to your feelings influences far more than your happiness or unhappiness. Your feelings are the voice of the collective unconscious attempting to heal itself.

According to Jung's theory—the time-honored concepts of psychiatrist Dr. Carl Gustav Jung, a contemporary of Freud's—the feeling function is *the ability to make evaluations and judgments based on values*. Feelings are your guides, barometers that enable you to say with integrity, "I like this" or "I don't like that," "I want this" or "I don't want that." Feelings are un-self-conscious, subjective, and experiential. They are always in *this moment*. They are an essential part of true awareness.

Getting in touch with your feeling function allows you to feel and express the purity of spirit that you had as a child. The reclaiming of the ability to listen to our feelings is not something that happens overnight, or in a flash of insight. It's accomplished only through practice. Day in, day out, we need to practice checking in with our feeling selves.

Ignoring your feelings prevents full awareness, which then leads you into the making of poor choices. If you don't check in with your feeling self, you may not see why you have an overriding desire to eat a giant bag of cookies in one sitting, and you might not be able to stop yourself. But once you have grown used to listening to your feelings, they'll trump your thoughts and beliefs, and your right path will show up as clearly as a lamp in the dark.

Listening to your body is very much a part of trusting your feelings. Learn to listen to your body's signals. And know that your body is not capable of error. It can only act wrongly when responding to a wrong thought. If you pay attention, you will find that your body is sending signals to your mind all the time. Have you ever agreed to do something that you knew was wrong? Did your body rebel as you tried to go ahead and do it anyway? Did you get butterflies in your stomach, feel like crying, or feel weak in the knees? Your body was giving you useful feedback.

Jung said that "neurosis is a substitute for legitimate suffering." Anxiety and depression both arise from us not being willing or able to face the truth of what we truly feel. Facing those feelings sets you free. You don't even have to do anything about them; you can just acknowledge them and allow them to be fully experienced in your body. They'll then dissolve into the next feeling, and the next, and the next. As you go on this ride from feeling to feeling, you will find that your choices are influenced. Those feelings will inform your food choices, your relationships, and your habits.

AWARENESS AND FOOD

To significantly improve your diet and your health requires both knowledge and practice: the knowledge of what happens to food once it enters the body and the effects it has on every dimension of health; and then the practice, the *translating* of this awareness into a good diet.

One reason diets don't work is because they are abstractions. Rather than accepting the latest ideology about "good" and "bad" kinds of food, we have to *love, respect,* and *understand* the food we eat. Don't just slavishly follow the advice of others! You will come to know, intuitively, which foods are best for you as you expand your ability to feel grateful for the food you eat; as you learn to thank the creatures that gave their lives to sustain you; as you approach eating not as something automatic and unaware, but as a consciously life-sustaining act.

We think of eating and drinking as mundane acts, but they are also sacred acts. They are archetypal, mystical rituals affirming life itself. They provide us with a daily connection to nature, our real mother. Each time we eat or drink, we have an opportunity to relate to and thank the vegetables, fish, birds, and other beings that gave their lives to feed us.

THE STRENGTH OF THE MIND

Once you become more aware of your feelings, you will be able to make the conscious choice to change the feelings in which you would rather not be stuck. You can use thought and the mind to do this.

So let's say you are stuck in feelings you wish to transform. The science of *psychoneuroimmunology* shows that our thoughts and feelings have many and potent effects on the workings of the body; it has also demonstrated that you can use your thoughts to alter your feelings and your physical self.

Thoughts alter the secretion and activity of hormones and neurotransmitters, the biochemical messengers that move information from cell to cell and from organ to organ. Once we become aware of our feelings, we can use this awareness to direct our minds, which can then feed back to alter our feelings in a positive way.

Let's say you're anxious and angry about the fight you had with your boss today. You've acknowledged this and sat with the feeling long enough, and you now want to change how you feel. Rather than eating a pint of ice cream or drinking four glasses of wine, you can use the power of your mind to see the pain this kind of reactive behavior will cost you. Then you are free to change your thoughts. "Maybe I should question the importance I put on my boss. It isn't important enough to make me destroy myself!" Instead of blindly scarfing down all that ice cream or wine, you can recognize what that desire is for and use the power of your mind to move to another level of consciousness, which will prevent you from acting on it. Jesus said to St. Thomas, "If you do not bring forth what is within you, what you do not bring forth will destroy you." Without awareness of what causes you to make bad choices, those choices will eventually destroy you.

Candace Pert was one of the first scientists to research the mind-body connection. Her fascinating book *Molecules of Emotion* describes her search for the molecules in the human nervous system that cause us to feel. In this book, she explores and articulates the relationships among body, mind, spirit, and emotion, and refines our understanding of reality itself and how we all cocreate it with our thoughts.

Some people worry that describing our feeling selves in terms of a few neurochemicals undermines the belief in a higher power, God or the soul. "If everything is just machinery, where does God or the soul fit in?" Pert answered that question after her scientific journey led her to a spiritual place, which she believes is the place where we achieve true health:

> Yes, we have a biochemical psychosomatic network run by intelligence, an intelligence that has no bounds and that is not owned by any individual but shared among all of us in a bigger network, the macrocosm to our microcosm, the "big psychosomatic network in the sky." And in this greater network of all humanity, all life, each of us is an individual node, each an access point into a larger intelligence. It is this shared connection that gives us our most profound sense of spirituality, making us feel connected, whole. (Candace Pert, *Molecules of Emotion*)

Spirituality and intelligence can go hand in hand—some would argue that they *must* do so—and together provide a strong foundation for positive change and a more healthful, soulful life.

THINK ABOUT THE REAL COST OF BAD CHOICES

If you keep making the same bad choices, you will keep getting the same bad results. If something isn't working, you've got to change it. How and where can you get the motivation? Here's the key: feel positive, recollect the best feelings you can recall, and associate them to the best outcome you are looking for. At the same time, think of the worst outcome and the stressful feeling it will bring. Feel them through and through, you will then have the experience of the emotional cost of not making healthful choices, avoiding disastrous, perhaps extremely painful consequences. We humans may not always go for the choice that's best for us, but we will do almost anything to avoid feelings of pain. You can use this human characteristic to your own advantage.

Physicians-authors Michael Roizen and Mehmet Oz are famous for giving patients actual sections of artery to feel with their fingers. They give them healthy arteries, which are flexible and soft, and have them compare these with atherosclerotic arteries that are calcified, lumpy, and bumpy. They also show the enlarged hearts of people with heart failure, the lungs of long-time smokers. These visual aids have dramatic impact on people who need to make better choices.

Poor choices will cause you to age very, very quickly; they could rob you of time with family and the freedom to move and enjoy life and find the ultimate meaning for your life. Do you have a round, fat belly that protrudes, even hangs over your belt? Is your waist measured around at the level of the belly button larger than the measurement around your hips? If it is larger, you are fat. Plain and simple. Your body is in danger. Beneath the surface of your belly, your viscera (guts) are laced with yellow, oily fat that is pouring inflammatory substances, cortisol and cholesterol, into your circulation. You need to know and be aware that you probably also have or soon will have high blood sugars, which will age and decay you at the cellular level with frightening speed.

Consider the price you will pay for eating that plate of cookies or that fried chicken. Think it's the last time you'll do it, so it's OK? Or you don't do this . . . *much?* Or that you *deserve* a treat because you've had a hard day? How many times have you told yourself these stories?

Pain is a terrific motivator—not even so much the threat of pain, but the actual experience. Hold on to that image of the consequences of your bad choice, and you'll find the strength to order that fruit salad or broiled fish instead.

The acquaintance who wrote to ask me about money could think about what will happen to him if he does not do what's necessary to get his finances in order. He might not be able to afford college for his kids, or retirement, or even to pay off his debts. Medical bills could bankrupt him. Once he has thought about these things and felt the fear and the pain this will cost him, he can begin to ask better questions and find ways to get what he wants.

As you move into healthier choices, when you make a mistake, or fall short, let it be a learning experience. Feel the pain of it. Acknowledge that you are harming yourself. Immediately start asking yourself better questions that can move the focus of your mind to new possibilities and better answers:

"How can I learn from this? How can I do better? What did I not do right? How can I make things the way I want them to be?"

You don't want to hurt. You want to be happy. This is *good*. Let this desire move you toward making better choices.

Close your eyes and think of a pink elephant standing right outside your window. You'll find yourself quite unable to *not* see that pachyderm in your mind, standing just outside those curtains, gazing in at you. It is amazing! All you need to do to change your reality is *change your focus*. Changing your reality might seem not to be easy, but it's fairly simple. And don't say, "Well, I'll *tryyyyyyy*." Children try. Adults *do*. Take action.

Don't talk, talk, and talk about your intentions or your frustrations or your shortcomings. Sit down with some paper and pen and write down your life plan. Write about what you want, where you are going. Don't complain, just envision where you want to go.

How much do you want to weigh? What kind of schedule do you want to keep, which charities do you want to volunteer to help? Where do you wish to travel? Who do you want to show that you love them unconditionally? Do you want to be alive and healthy without pain—one, five, ten, or twenty years from now?

How do you want to die? Where?

How will you be laid to rest? What will your eulogy be like?

Your legacy?

CHAPTER TWO

Stay in Touch

DESPITE ALL OUR technological advances and the one-hundred-plus cable channels that we watch in our home entertainment centers, the subject that most interests us has not changed since the theater arts first began millennia ago in ancient Greece: interpersonal relationships.

When we touch one another, atoms bounce back and forth between the skins of both people. When we touch an object, we leave some of our atoms on its surface, and some of its atoms stay on our skin. A newborn baby is made of star stuff, which has existed for billions of years. Each of us is made from this stuff, which is continually recycled through our bodies and objects over time. The food we eat becomes our bodies, and the thoughts we think create our bodies as well. All parts of ourselves—including our thoughts, beliefs, and feelings—are interacting.

The majority of television programming is about relationships. Talk shows give advice about how to get into one, how to sustain one, and how to get out of one. Reality shows explore the ways in which people interact under elaborately orchestrated circumstances that hardly resemble real life. Situation comedies find the humor in relationships while dramas pull at our heartstrings with relationship-related ups and downs. The news also focuses increasingly on relationships with their human interest stories, rather than reporting the events in a straightforward way.

TV is all about relationships, but mostly the wrong relationships. It is about relating to an idea or image of how the other person or the self should be.

THE HUMAN PROJECTOR

Carl Jung believed that everything about ourselves that we are not conscious of is projected on to someone else. We naturally assume that the world is as we see it and that other people are what we imagine and assume them to be. Therefore, we see in other people or in things (such as foods or institutions) our worst features—and our best, most undeveloped, wonderful features.

We project our own beauty and greatness into other people or things: movie stars, celebrities, plays, books, foods, politicians. We may also project our own beauty and greatness on to institutions: restaurants, religions, sects, political parties. People can become junkies with anything—whether the projection is wonderful ("that Oprah Winfrey is so amazing; I wish I could be like her!") or awful ("those right-wingers are so evil, and I'll spend the next hour telling you exactly why!").

You can get just as hooked on something you see as bad and evil as on something you see as beautiful and good. Anyone who has spent any amount of time crusading against anything knows this. This is because you are projecting something dark, from your shadow side, out of yourself on to something else. You are inexorably drawn to that projection, whether it's good or bad, because it is a part of you.

We also can project into foods, animals, and things, seeing them as wonderful or terrible. What is projected is an image of our own shadow side or unrecognized gifts, an idea associated with an emotional content that is pleasurable or painful, pleasant or unpleasant.

What is good about projection is that just as we project things, we can take them back. To do this, we must become consciously aware that it is not *that* which is beautiful or ugly; it is we ourselves who are beautiful or ugly. Projection works like a two-way mirror. The other person, entity, or organization is a reflection of our own unacknowledged face. It is a blurry mirror, where it is not easy to tell who's who.

Withdrawing projections can be painful and will not happen overnight but is fundamental in the process of becoming aware and conscious. Owning the part of yourself that is being projected on to foods, other people, or things will transform your relationship with these foods, people, or things. If you do not become aware of what you are projecting, you cannot have a relationship that is conscious, fulfilling, or healthy.

Becoming conscious is a continuous process of assimilating what was previously unknown to our ego. It is a progressive awakening to why we do what we do. Being conscious is not a question of IQ or about any other measure of how smart you are or how many degrees you have. It is a completely subjective phenomenon; it depends on how much we know about ourselves.

The opinions of the radio and television pedants are their own projections. This is why I'm never surprised to see an anti-prostitution crusader caught with his pants down, or to see anti-drug crusaders and to addicted to drugs. This is exactly what *should* happen; their crusades and opinions are projections of their own shadow sides.

Still, we look to these mouthpieces of our society because we are so unconscious that we think we need their opinions—which are really their projections—because they seem so sure and real. The key to changing the world is for all of us to recognize that we are projecting and to own our own perceptions and shadow sides. Then we can be in real relationship with one another. This is the beginning of needed change in the world. The collective unconsciousness has to wake up. Otherwise, change will not happen.

Whatever aspects of ourselves we are not conscious of, we see in someone else. If we are not aware that we are projecting images, are we having "relationships" with others at all? Not really, we only relate to ourselves when we do not see that we are projecting.

You cannot truly have a right relationship with anybody unless you are aware of yourself. Without that awareness, the other is only an image you project from yourself. Images don't relate outside the realm of fantasy. We tend to think that what we see in ourselves is in others and that the same motives are everywhere. What is pleasurable for us is pleasurable for others. This is why people always want to correct others, why they find fault with one another and blame one another. We are projecting: seeing in others what is in ourselves. So what needs most correcting in the whole world is . . . ourselves.

These projections must be faced head-on. How can this be done? You can start by

- no longer complaining about anyone or anything. Not even your discontent! Complaints are projections of your inner discontent. To project that on to something or someone outside of you is to give up control over it. You don't have to do that. Claim responsibility, and *voila!*—you also claim power and control.
- no longer worshipping anybody or anything. Rather than worshipping the skinny people or the artists or the junk food or the celebrity, realize *those qualities you have worshipped are all in you*. That's right; you are as delicious as junk food, as gorgeous as the skinny movie star, as creative as the artist.

To truly relate and to truly love, we need to know a person or thing as it really is. This is human-sized love, and it is the only and best kind of love available to us.

If the characters on your favorite program embraced total acceptance of the reality of the other characters, rather than holding them up to made-up ideas of how they should be . . . well, there wouldn't be much drama to speak of, and your favorite actors would soon be out of work. But TV is not real life. You can enter a place of total acceptance of the people with whom you choose to relate in your own life. Drama is fun on television, but in your real life, it's a burdensome distraction from optimization.

When it comes to your relationship with food, the same concepts apply to the media blitz versus the reality of a life made up of good choices. People who talk about food and give advice in the media talk about ideas: about supplements, exercises, "super-foods" that will magically transform your body. None of these ideas easily translate into a real, personal relationship with food and health.

If you want to optimize your life, you will need to stop allowing yourself to be manipulated by the media. You don't need it. It's only a relationship with an image, and it stands in the way of your observing reality without judgment.

Having real, right relationships, unlike watching TV programs, requires awareness. Until we can relate clearly without presuppositions about what the other should be, we can't have real relationships—not with other people, with ourselves, or with the food we eat. And those real relationships are the key to making healthful changes for life.

Wrong relationship is based on projected images, not reality. It is about wanting what you don't have, about expecting the images you have of others to give you what your image demands and wants, and then feeling like a victim when you don't get it. From wrong relationships spring need, fear, doubt, anger, and competition.

Right relationship is based on conscious psychological relationship between conscious people. It is being able to see what is real and truly in front of us, not images; is about taking responsibility for our own choices and accepting others as they are, in this moment, knowing you cannot change them. You can do this with your spouse ("the reality is that my husband is never, ever, going to pick up his socks"), with yourself (usually, some variation on "I'm not perfect, and I accept and love myself"), or with your food ("the reality is that a bacon double cheeseburger is poison to my body"). Relating consciously to the truth creates love, trust, acceptance, gratitude, and compassion.

We can approach our journey toward better health as a series of wrong relationships being righted. Illiteracy replaced with literacy. As you ask the following questions in assessing your relationships, ask yourself how you might be sabotaging your attempts to move into a more healthful lifestyle.

What Kind of Relationship Do You Have with Your Body?

Have you ever questioned the relationship you have with your body? If you're like many people who battle weight problems, feelings of not being attractive, or having a chronic disease, you are projecting dark, ugly images on to your body, and that's what you see. You may feel angry at your body, feeling as though it is ugly and has betrayed you. That you are afraid of being powerless to change course. Becoming conscious of this will begin to transform this relationship.

What Kind of Relationship Do You Have with Yourself?

Do you love yourself as passionately as you would like to be loved by others? Are you trapped in self-hatred? Or are you somewhere in between? How does your relationship with yourself affect the feeding and nurturing that you give yourself? What kind of things do you say to yourself that you would never say to another person? Can you see how you might treat yourself better—as a valued friend, or a beloved member of your own family?

What Kind of Relationships Do You Have with Other People?

Are your relationships with others sources of joy, personal growth, and contentment, or are they hotbeds of unpleasantness filled with unresolved conflict and stress? Do you tell lies to maintain relationships, relationships that are unhealthy and conflicted? Do you devote yourself to pleasing others and derive your sense of self-worth from how well you do so? Do you use relationships to create dramas that distract you from the issues you don't want to address?

Cultivate an awareness of when you are holding an unrealistic image and trying to fit your mate (or prospective mate, parent, sibling, child, or friend) into it rather than acknowledging, respecting, and dealing with the flesh-and-blood person sitting in front of you.

What Is Your Relationship with Food?

Food is one of our last remaining links to the natural world, a world from which most of us have become increasingly removed. Food is energy, and your relationship to food is your relationship to energy. As long as you relate to food in an unconscious, unaware way, it is not possible for you to break the cycle of poor eating habits and make good choices. Enlightened eating—right relationship with your food, chosen with awareness—gives you a whole different kind of energy.

Do you have an addiction to junk food, relying on its intense, addictive flavors to take you out of your meaningless state and all its loneliness and pain? Junk foods taste good, and they even make you feel good—at least, they give you a different kind of energy. For a while, after you eat this kind of food, you feel on top of the world, despite twinges of guilt for feeding yourself something so unhealthy. Then, that short burst of energy fades, and you go back for more of the same kind of food. The guilt you feel for eating junk augments your need for a "pick-me-up" that often comes in the form of more junk.

It's like that romantic relationship you had that you knew was all wrong, even destructive, but you didn't have the grounded awareness that would enable you to stay away.

As you learn more about how foods interact energetically in your body, you will drop your unhealthy patterns. You will associate unhealthy foods with pain, and you will stick with food that nourishes, empowers, and energizes you. Knowing how unhealthy foods hurt you and how healthy foods enrich your life will help you to make good choices and stay with a moderate approach.

Make a commitment to bettering your relationships with food, with other people, and then with yourself. Until this happens, all your intentions are just talk.

Decide to commit to seeking good energy and giving good energy. Do so fully, with all your heart, soul, and mind.

LOVE IS AT THE HEART OF ALL RELATIONSHIPS

Whether you are relating to yourself, your food, or other people, the keys to making those relationships loving are the same.

Love yourself. If we are all made in the image of God, what could possibly be so wrong with you? Look inside. See your value. You are a child of

God—you've got it all! Being comfortable with yourself is the first big step to healthier relationship. When you rely on another person, object, or food to "complete" you or cause you to feel self-love, you are not in a truly loving relationship.

Love . . . just love! Too often, we want to be loved before we give love or before we can love ourselves. It doesn't work this way. Open your heart; pour love out of yourself. You can give a limitless amount of love, and once you recognize this, it will come back to you in even greater quantities. As the *Course in Miracles* tells us, "To have, give all to all." If you feel that self-love is beyond your grasp, enlist the aid of a skilled therapist or enroll yourself in a spiritual practice to help you overcome whatever is in the way.

Love is irreducible and abundant. Like spiritual experience, it defies description. This love is intelligent; this love is energy; this love moves everything and makes everything possible. Some call this love God or believe that it springs from God.

Take a moment and allow yourself to feel love and only love in the center of your chest—love for the trees, the ants, the pebbles, and all of nature. Remember that you are a part of that beauty. This will not be easy at first, and you might feel uncomfortable as your ego chatters away in the background with a never-ending stream of doubts, questions, and criticisms. Acknowledge the chatter in a friendly way . . . and keep feeling love.

LOVE VS. FEAR

Love is the "glue" of the universe, connecting all people. It is a field, outside of which everything appears fragmented. There is only one catch, which lives in the minds of most people and cannot coexist with the kind of love described here. It's a little thing called fear.

I refer not to the kind of fear that elicits a physiological and constructive "fight-or-flight" response, enabling you to act quickly and avoid physical harm. Instead, I refer here to the kind of fear mediated by thought, passed down through generations, that stands in the way of love. This fear is founded in ways of describing and thinking about the world that are passed down and taught. It springs from what we have been taught in the past and has no real footing in the present. To make this distinction, try to imagine what a wild animal might be afraid of. (Domesticated pets can be as neurotic as their owners.) They don't waste energy fearing that which is not a threat to their safety.

When an antelope is being chased by a lion, it doesn't feel fear as an emotion; it feels a surge of adrenaline that enables it to bound to safety. The antelope doesn't sit around worrying that a lion is going to come after it; and once it escapes, it doesn't sit around thinking, "Whoa! That was a close one!" If it needs to fight, it fights to the death and doesn't think about the outcome.

Imagine that you have narrowly avoided being in an automobile accident. You might spend hours reliving and thinking about the incident. Even days later, anger and fear might keep causing your stomach to knot, your muscles to tense. The hormones that elicited the fight-or-flight response—cortisol and norepinephrine—continue to be secreted by your adrenal glands, raising your blood pressure, increasing your heart and respiratory rates, disrupting your digestion, and making your thinking less clear.

As you remain trapped in that moment of fear, you accelerate your body's aging, increase your appetite (particularly cravings for sugars and fat), and bring on tension and body aches. All these things make sickness and injury more likely.

Holding a grudge or nursing a psychic wound by thinking about past harms or future risks is harmful to you. This is how anxiety is created: by relating to an image from the past or future, not to the reality of the present moment.

When you come from fear, you might think, "That jerk that cut me off ought to die a horrible death—twice!" But when you come from love, you might have thoughts like "That person might be in a hurry for a good reason," "Thank goodness no one was hurt," or "I've done the same thing to other drivers without meaning to . . . now I know how the other person feels!"

This same transformation can be applied to losing weight: "I want to lose weight because I hate myself like this," becomes "I want to lose weight because I love myself, because I am passionate about life and want to enjoy every moment."

When you come from love rather than fear, a statement like "I don't want to say what I mean because I am afraid I will make so-and-so angry," becomes "I'm going to tell the truth as gently and kindly as I can."

To give love is to empower another person, to "charge" them in a way that dissolves fear. In centuries past, it was the king's due to receive the energy of all his subjects. He could also look you in the eye and bless you, giving that energy back; or he could give you the *malocue*, or "bad eye," and sap you of your energy. The truth is that we all have the power to bless or give the *malocue* to others. Choose love and empower others, and you are in the field of abundance. Love is joyful sacrifice. It's limitless, and the more you give, the more you get in return.

Love rejoices only in truth. It protects, hopes, trusts, and perseveres. In love we are powerful. In love the need to attack or defend dissolves.

"I want to love," you might think, "but I am so angry." Anger and fear are two sides of the same coin. The angry person is the fearful one. This is where forgiveness enters the picture.

WHEN STRESS STRIKES, PAUSE AND DEFUSE

Reacting from anger and fear creates a huge conflict. Awareness flies out the window, and you waste all kinds of time engaged in a battle that doesn't have to happen. Here are a few ways to cope with the emotions that can come up in the context of relationships.

Stress-Coping Techniques: A Checklist

All these methods have been found to delay the aging process, support immune system function, and enhance well-being:

- Aromatherapy: Try keeping a bottle of oil of lavender around and rub some on a pulse point on your neck or your wrists when you are feeling stressed. It will soothe and refresh you.

- Breath work/meditation: Sit with eyes closed in a quiet place and breathe deeply until you feel calm. Throughout the day, remind yourself to breathe deeply and slowly.
- Exercise: Sweat the stress out!
- Get organized: Disorganization is a major cause of stress in modern life. If you can never find anything and you know your life's a mess, set aside a couple of days and make organization your top priority.
- Hands-on work: Garden, knit, build, paint, tinker.
- Maintain awareness: Notice the physical signs of stress in your body and acknowledge them when they arise. "Oh, my shoulders are tensing up. My forehead feels tense too." Then breathe deeply and exhale the tension away.
- Massage: An hour's massage once a week is a terrific stress-reducing gift to give yourself. Or buy a book on massage and learn with your partner.
- Music: Listen to music that soothes or inspires you.
- Religious or spiritual ritual: Meditating, praying, chanting, and fasting are all rituals that have sustained people through tough times. Recent research shows that these practices can extend life and improve health.
- Laughter: Find a way to laugh, hard—not just a chuckle or a giggle, but a belly laugh that leaves you breathless!
- Sacred spot: Set aside a special place in your home for relaxation and spiritual practices. Deck it out with the colors and objects that most appeal to you. Spend time there whenever you need to defuse or recharge.
- Visualization: Close your eyes and picture something beautiful and serene.
- Yoga: An ancient way to maintain a strong, flexible body and an open, loving mind.

Bad ways to deal with stress include taking drugs (alcohol included), bingeing on food, creating unnecessary drama, watching television, surfing the Internet, and directing anger/judgment/blame/shame toward others.

Don't make stress reduction just another source of stress: "Oh, damn, I didn't meditate today!" Instead, integrate stress reduction into your life as something you do naturally whenever your feelings tell you it's time.

ANGER AND FORGIVENESS

Forgiveness is a key to happiness. It releases us from guilt and fear and is the greatest gift we can give to ourselves and to others. Love can only be when we let go of fear. The mind that is not forgiving is full of fear and has no room for love; it remains sad, angry, and resentful without hope of peace and joy. The unforgiving person is torn with doubt, confused about itself and all he sees, afraid and angry, and in despair.

When you forgive, you step out of the struggle into love and clarity.

Whomever you judge or dislike, forgive. This is a big step toward releasing yourself from any fear that lingers in your mind and from the stress that comes from being judgmental and angry.

And don't forget to forgive *yourself*. Instead of making excuses, blaming your misdeeds on others, or saying that you couldn't help it because you have this or that psychological disorder, take responsibility (with responsibility comes power after all), forgive yourself and move on.

HEALTHY RELATIONSHIPS OPTIMIZE YOUR LIFE

Much scientific research supports the idea that being an active partner in a healthy, supportive intimate relationship will extend your life. A study from the University of Michigan showed that older people who reported giving emotional or other kinds of support to their spouses lived longer than those who reported receiving support. A study from Columbia University reported similar findings, showing that spouses who reported being the main source of emotional support for their partners were much less likely to die during the course of the study.

A study by Spanish researchers found that elderly people who cohabit with others live longer. Contact with neighbors and the community at large also promotes longer life. Community and service involvement is vital in old age—to age well. This usually involves a large network of relationships. All this has been firmly linked to longevity, vitality, productivity, and good health in a number of long prospective studies.

The question remains: do those who gain health and longevity through relationship know something the rest of us don't? Do they understand how to relate to others in a healthy way? Most likely. Some find this easy, having been loved and related so well by their parents or within other important relationships. Others have not been so lucky.

Even though our ways of relating might be leading to enormous conflict, we rarely question those ways because they are so much a part of us. When you attempt to change the way in which you relate to others, you can feel strange, false, wrong because you've always done it the other way, and probably, so did your parents.

Some people have difficult relationships characterized by constant fighting. This is worse than a waste of time—it takes years off your life; ages you prematurely; and leads to depression, anxiety, and unnecessary tension. Unlike what many people on talk shows seem to believe, the answer is not for the other person to finally see things your way. The answer is far more complex than this, but also far simpler: to find ways to relate to others that are consistently loving, accepting, compassionate, and peaceful.

That's right; lose the drama. It is only a distraction! Instead of heightening the conflict, step back from it. If you have the energy, put love into the equation and see how things change. Tell yourself or your partner what you are feeling and what you need. Avoid blaming anyone, *including yourself.* You are responsible for knowing and then asking for what you need. Don't expect your partner to know what you need, even if you think it ought to be totally obvious. Tell *yourself exactly* what you need in clear, concise, totally honest language, if you're relating to yourself only.

If you do not have anything good to say about the person you are relating to (or yourself, or even to the food you're eating), then don't say anything, but look for something good to say. There is always something good to notice and remark upon in everyone, in everything, always something for which you can be thankful. Instead of "You're hurting me, and that means you're bad, terrible, and wrong, it's your entire fault," deal with the problem, not the person or thing that might have caused it. Own your part in it too.

"I am not getting what I need," tell yourself or the other person. "How do I get what I need?" Enlist their help and support in getting what you need, whether it's more time to yourself, more time together, a less stressful job, more sex, less sex, a different kind of sex, or less junk food in the pantry. You might not get what you need, but your chances are far better if you speak out about it.

Tell the truth about everything and tell it always. This does not mean telling your partner that she looks fat in those pants or that he is not actually as good a dancer as he believes himself to be. It means speaking plainly about what *you* are feeling, about what *you* want.

There is no such thing as dishonest communication. If you are not being honest, you are not communicating. Make your needs known but release the expectation that they will be met. And be honest with yourself when you hear yourself saying one thing but doing something else. (We all do it.) Acknowledge it and change your behavior.

Don't blame anything or anyone when things go wrong. In nonviolent communication (NVC), a method of communicating feelings and needs to others, we are advised to avoid judgment, anger, blame, and shame (JABS) when relating to self or others. This is a good guideline for any relationship, including the one you have with the food you eat.

Keep practicing getting in touch and with sharing your feelings. If you are having a dispute with your spouse or struggling internally with an issue, stop defending yourself and accusing others. Simply say, "I am feeling very angry right now," or "I am feeling hurt," or "When you say I am stupid, I feel angry and hurt." On the other hand, if you say, "You are hurting me," or "It's all so-and-so's fault," or "Oh, yeah? You think I'm wrong? Well, you're a stupid [insert a stream of expletives here]," you are projecting your own dark shadow material. Do you see the difference? In the first way, you take responsibility and state the truth; in the second, your dark shadow makes you feel like a victim, inflicted upon and out of control, as you attempt to manipulate the other by making statements designed to inflict guilt and wield control.

Don't blame the nacho cheese corn chips for being unhealthy *and* delicious. Don't be angry at the giant food manufacturing conglomerate for creating that fabulous advertising that equates nacho cheese dust on your fingertips with fun and attractive friends. You are aware that the giant food manufacturing conglomerates are using us for profit and transforming human beings into consumers. You are aware that you don't want to consume what is toxic to your one and only body, the vessel of your soul. And you are fully responsible for getting your own healthy needs met. Those needs, quite simply, do not include that bag of chips.

As you work toward consciousness and awareness, you will develop new, clear, honest, direct ways of relating. Notice: How are others beginning to respond to you? Are you getting into fewer conflicts with your spouse? Do you feel more energy as love and contentment? Are you more relaxed? Do you laugh more? Do you feel more loving and loved? Stay with the *now*! Enjoy. Do not *do*; just be!

RESPECT YOURSELF, RESPECT OTHERS

Respect yourself and the people in your life. Do this by always pouring loving energy into any situation. Surprise your partner with little gifts, notes, and other forms of loving attention. Help him or her with tasks and always be on the lookout for ways you can offer love and support. Appreciate and respect life energy from the foods you eat, a gift of sustenance straight from the bosom of Mother Earth.

Do the same for your home, your spouse and children, and at your work. Respect becomes easy with self-awareness because self-awareness includes the understanding that we are all one. We are also all one with our surroundings; when you take good care of your surroundings, you are giving yourself the gift of life and joy because any separation of you from those surroundings is an illusion. As you learn to cohabit respectfully with other beings, the food you eat, and the objects that surround you, you will feel more centered, clear, orderly, and full of love.

As you become more and more impeccable with your words, it will become easier to honor the commitments you make to yourself and others. Your respect for yourself will shine through to those with whom you relate, setting an example of what it is to embrace what is life-giving and to stay away from all that takes our energy and injures the body and soul.

Commit to live a healthy, long life with the purpose of becoming conscious, aware, wise, and full of loving energy that easily flows out to other people.

Vanity, in any form, indicates that you feel unworthy and that you are projecting your self-worth to others as you attempt to impress them, be accepted, and be liked. This is a huge waste of energy. Be aware of this. Withdraw that projection and see yourself as the beautiful person that you are. Look at your body, your face; realize that you are unique and bring love to that image.

You can feel energized, content, and at peace just the way you are; on the other hand, keeping yourself up, wearing clothing you love, and keeping your hair and skin looking their best is a great gift to give yourself. When you are doing it for yourself and not to satisfy your vanity, it will make you feel good. Look at nature. The flowers want to look the best they can. The birds too! Preening and displaying and attracting goes on all the time in the natural world, and we humans are very much a part of nature whether we like it or not. We honor our bond with nature when we take especially good care of ourselves and do what we can to make ourselves beautiful. But if you're a canary, be the most beautiful canary you can be. Don't pretend to be a falcon.

THE NEXT STEP

This book is a journey. It may be the most important one you will ever take, and one that we all need to take sooner or later if we wish to have a second chance at life. The information in these pages will help you to have the time and vitality to live your life to the hilt. You can live the life you were born to live, holding the tensions of culture, religion, family, and history.

All the information in this book has been used in my journey through life. I feel confident that it will transform you into a health-literate individual—and to know that any effective and lasting improvements you make in your health will ultimately come to give you that second chance, providing you with the chronos time you may need for your evolution into higher levels of consciousness and awareness where you can then live in kayros time. You might call this *attending to the soul*.

From this point forward, this book will shift into a much more scientifically oriented space. You will learn a great deal of information about how foods affect your body at the cellular level, about how hormones operate and how they can be balanced, and about other matters corporeal. This might seem curious after all this talk about spirit and soul, but many of our greatest scientists were deeply spiritual individuals who knew that without attention to soul and spirit, even the most brilliant scientific discoveries ring hollow.

As Albert Einstein said:

> *You will hardly find one among the profounder sort of scientific minds without a religious feeling of his own. But it is different from the religiosity of the naïve man. For the latter, God is a being from whose care one hopes to benefit and whose punishment one fears; a sublimation of a feeling similar to that of a child for its father, a being to whom one stands, so to speak, in a* personal *relation, however deeply it may be tinged with awe.*
>
> *But the scientist is possessed by the sense of universal causation . . . His religious feeling takes the form of a rapturous amazement at the harmony of natural law, which reveals an intelligence of such superiority that, compared with it, all the systematic thinking and acting of human beings is an utterly insignificant reflection.*

CHAPTER THREE

The Biology of Aging

I HOPE THAT by now you have grasped that aging is as much about the mind as it is about the body. If you think of yourself as an old fart, congratulations—you are an old fart!

Of course, aging brings about certain physical changes. But still, within the framework of those changes—which go all the way down to the level of DNA—we have a lot of wiggle room. Our beliefs, our thoughts, our self-talk, our relationships, our eating habits, and our other lifestyle choices can do much to mitigate the changes associated with aging.

Let's take one of my patients, Jeremy, as an example. Like me, Jeremy is a physician, and he is powerfully invested in staying as youthful and energetic as he can. At sixty-four he has no desire to stop practicing medicine, which is his greatest passion. Where so many people his age suffer from high blood pressure and cholesterol, worsening eyesight, creeping weight gain, falling bone density, and rising insulin and blood sugar levels, he does not. After years of following my prescriptions, he has become highly food literate and judiciously uses hormone replacement and nutritional supplements. He has terrific health to show for it, including

- a great sex life,
- insulin and blood sugar levels well below problem ranges,
- an LDL cholesterol level below 100 and an HDL above 45,
- skin that remains smooth and supple,
- a perfect ratio of fat to muscle (about 18 percent body fat),
- no signs of "senior moments" or diminished energy.

I have a lot of patients like Jeremy. All this is within your grasp with the right awareness and information.

WHAT WILL CHANGE, NO MATTER WHAT

Here are some body changes you can all but count on as you get older. Depending on your genetic makeup and the environmental pleasures and insults you've experienced, these changes can be extensive or mild.

- Farsightedness
- Graying of hair
- Hardening of the arteries (stiffening of the artery walls, which is not the same thing as atherosclerosis, where fatty plaque builds up in the arterial lining)
- Loss of high-tone hearing
- Loss of skin elasticity

Everything else is much more under your control. If you go to a doctor who tells you that anything in the following list is an inevitable part of growing older, you might want to find yourself a new doctor:

- Adult-onset diabetes
- Arthritis
- Cancer
- Decrease in digestive function that leads to indigestion and bowel problems
- Decrease in memory
- Diminished intelligence
- Dramatic loss of physical flexibility and endurance
- Falling bone mineral density
- Heart attack
- High blood pressure
- Loss of libido or sexual function
- Prostate enlargement
- Rising body mass index (ratio of height to weight)
- Rising cholesterol count

While not everyone can avoid all these conditions, most people can avoid most of them or keep them at bay until very late in life. And if and when they do happen, the intensity of the condition can be lessened with the right interventions.

THEORIES OF AGING

Some organisms don't age, but live on as long as they have access to an energy source. Single-celled organisms, for example, divide to create identical offspring and keep on making more clones of themselves until the food runs out.

This is the root of the aging problem: Any organism that reproduces through sexual means—where the union of germ cells (sperm and egg) creates an entirely new being—will age and die. Science refers to this as the disposable soma theory of aging: that investing life energy in the creation of germ cells leaves less energy for maintaining the body (soma). Every cell in our bodies is programmed to self-destruct because we reproduce sexually. The price we pay for sex is death.

This is, fundamentally, why we age; the remainder of this chapter explains some of the ideas science has come up with about how we age.

In this chapter, I hope to educate you about the ways in which the body ages. This information will help you to fully grasp the chapters that follow, which cover specific ways to intervene in the physical aging process and prevent chronic disease. As you learn about the various scientific theories about why we age, keep in mind that they are all likely to play a part; no one theory explains it all. Some are more compelling or more important than others.

Using this knowledge to slow the aging process and prevent disease will allow you to chase your dreams, manifest your genius, and be of help in the world . . . with fewer interruptions from a body that is falling apart.

HOW WE AGE: A FEW THEORIES

The relationships among genes, environment, and perception are orchestrated by complex systems of hormones, neurotransmitters, and other molecular messengers that can either create or destroy our cells, tissues, organs, and bodies.

Our bodies spend the first thirty years or so of life producing more cells than are destroyed by regular wear and tear. Hormones, neurotransmitters, and genes collaborate to transform a newborn infant into an adult. Cells are built from fatty acids and proteins, tissues from cells, organs from tissues. Fuel enters the body as food and is either "burned" or stored in fat, muscle, or liver. In the preteen or teen years, sexual maturity is reached, with hormones and neurotransmitters orchestrating all these processes as well.

After the age of thirty or so, the efficiency of physiological functions begins to decline. Think of the natural rate of aging as a bell curve, with the centermost point falling at about the third decade of life. What we're trying to do with Age Optimization is push the top of that curve to the right so that we only see a real acceleration of aging when our lives are almost over.

Humans have been trying to forestall aging and avoid death ever since we gave up on finding the fountain of youth. Most of the approximately three hundred theories of aging have attempted to explain exactly what goes on at the cellular level to cause us to age, in hopes of pointing the way to possible interventions. Following are eleven of the most compelling of the aging theories, all of which probably are at least partly accurate. Each gives us clues about interventions that can slow physical aging—interventions covered in this book.

Wear and Tear Theory

This was one of the first theories of aging, introduced in the latter part of the nineteenth century. It says that the cells and organs of the body sustain damage from environmental and dietary toxins, ultraviolet solar radiation, and various physical and emotional stresses. A youthful body is able to repair the damage caused by wear and tear, but an aging body loses its capacity to bounce back.

To reduce wear and tear, protect yourself from the sun, find ways to minimize the impact of stress, and don't do anything to excess. Eating less junk and less food in general (see caloric restriction theory) will reduce toxic load; so will attention to keeping your diet and surroundings as green and organic as possible.

Waste Accumulation Theory

Just like humanity, it seems that individual cells make more trash than they can get rid of. Cellular waste materials eventually build up, gumming up the works of cells and causing their demise. Laboratory studies have shown that cells containing more metabolic wastes divide more slowly than cells that contain less.

Eating less, eating better, and drinking adequate water (at least eight eight-ounce glasses a day) will help reduce accumulation of cellular "junk."

Neuroendocrine Theory

Age-related changes in the body's production of growth hormone, thyroid hormone, the sex hormones (estrogen, progesterone, and testosterone), cortisol, DHEA, and melatonin strongly impact our bodies at the cellular level. The effect of one hormone falling out of balance cascades throughout the body and causes other hormones to do the same.

Modern medicine can safely rebalance hormones so their levels resemble those of a younger person. With the hormone activity of a person half your age, you can come close to maintaining the cellular metabolic activity of a person of that age.

While you might not need hormone replacement to remain healthy as you age, it certainly will not hurt as long as you follow specific guidelines. The science of hormone replacement has come a lot further than you might think, with all the bad press it has received in recent years. Chapters Six through Eight of this book give guidance about safe, effective hormone replacement.

Genetic Control Theory

Each person's unique genetic code predetermines much about that person: eye color, hair color, body type, and vulnerability to certain life-threatening diseases, such as cancer or heart disease. In most cases, genetic vulnerability explains only a fraction of the incidence of diseases commonly related to aging.

Genes are a blueprint that can be worked within. If you have a genetic predisposition to a certain disease, it might still be the thing that does you in, but you can still do a lot in terms of prevention or postponement of that illness with healthy lifestyle choices.

Telomerase Theory

Scientists at the Geron Corporation, a biotechnology research firm in Menlo Park, California, discovered small "tags" of nucleic acids (the building blocks of DNA) named telomeres. Telomeres act as a sort of aging clock for cells, allowing them to divide only a certain number of times before they die.

Telomeres are chunks of DNA that lie at the ends of chromosomes. Each time a cell divides to yield new cells, its telomeres shrink. When the telomeres are completely gone, cell division chips away at the chromosome itself, and the chromosome malfunctions. The cell is no longer able to do its job and eventually dies.

We know that telomere shortening is accelerated by stress. Researchers Elissa Epel and Elizabeth Blackburn of the University of California at San Francisco (UCSF) measured the telomere shortening of thirty-nine mothers who had a child with autism or cerebral palsy and nineteen mothers with normal children. The researchers found that the longer a woman had been caring for a sick child, the shorter her telomeres. Here's the really interesting part: the more intense the mother's perception of her stress, the more her telomeres had shortened. The women who were worst off had telomeres whose lengths were the sizes of people ten years older.

The hormone cortisol, which is secreted in response to stress, has been found to damage telomeres. If high stress equals shorter telomeres, then reducing the impact of stress should have the opposite effect.

Hayflick Limit Theory

Cellular biologists Hayflick and Moorehead demonstrated that lung, skin, muscle, and heart cells divide approximately fifty times in the course of their life spans. When overfed, these cells divided much more rapidly, making their fifty divisions in only one year. When underfed, cells divide up to three times more slowly. Cells approaching their growth limit have more degenerative changes than younger cells.

Caloric Restriction Theory

This theory builds on the Hayflick limit. Restricting calories to about 30 percent less than one would eat if one had unlimited access to food extends life span. This is true for most species, from tiny segmented worms to rodents to human beings. Less food means less wear and tear, less free-radical stress, reduced inflammation, fewer toxic substances from foods, and less fat.

Eating less than you want is not easy. By doing so, you are going against your deeply ingrained instinct to eat today, for tomorrow you might have less food—the case for much of human history. The next best alternative is to eat highly nutrient-rich foods so the body gets the highest possible amounts of vitamins, minerals, and corollary nutrients per calorie eaten.

Rate of Living Theory

This theory of aging correlates metabolic rate to life span and was introduced by German physiologist Max Rubner in 1908. It is the medical equivalent to the adage "Live fast, die young." For example, a tiny mouse, which has a very high heart rate, can only live for a few years while a human being can live to one hundred or more. Chimpanzees have a metabolic rate somewhat faster than humans, with their maximum life span being around twenty-seven years.

This rule does not apply in all cases—some species' metabolic rates are poor predictors of their life span—but relating these two variables makes sense. The higher the metabolic rate, the greater the wear and tear and waste accumulation.

Stress increases metabolic rate, accelerating the aging process. Reduce stress, reduce metabolic rate, and live a longer and happier life. This might run counter to the idea that you should raise your metabolic rate to lose weight; but really, if you consider the big picture, you are far better off with less stress and strain. Just eat less food and better food and be physically active and fit, and you won't have to worry so much about "burning off" all those excess calories!

Cross-linkage Theory

Collagen is the "glue" of the body, the connective tissue that keeps us all in one piece. When we are young, collagen has few cross-linkages where collagen molecules bind to one another. Un-cross-linked collagen remains soft and pliable, giving us flexible blood vessel walls, smooth skin, and supple joints. As we age, collagen cross-linkages increase, causing tissues to become stiff. The passage of nutrients between cells is also thought to be hampered by increased collagen cross-linkage, which decreases the flexibility and permeability of tissues.

Is there a way to reduce collagen cross-linkage? Yes—by reducing the processes of glycation, oxidation, and inflammation, which is covered in detail below and in chapters to come.

Immunity Theories

Some theories of aging focus on the decrease in immune system functioning. With age, the immune system loses some of its ability to fight off infectious agents and can become overreactive, causing allergies and autoimmune disease.

Healthful eating and regular exercise, as described in this book, will enhance and balance immune function. So will healthy relationships and stress-reducing, awareness-raising practices. All this will be covered in chapters to come.

THE BIG THREE: INFLAMMATION, OXIDATION, AND GLYCATION

These theories of aging, unlike some of the previous ones, have been strongly validated by science. Understanding them will give you a lot of power to minimize the less positive effects of aging.

Oxidation, inflammation, and glycation are all interrelated. Let's start with what is probably the most important of the three: oxidation.

Oxidation: Free-Radical Free-for-All

Within nearly every type of body cell are organelles—"little organs"—called mitochondria. The mitochondria are responsible for metabolism. They take in glucose (the most basic component of carbohydrates) and fatty acids (the most basic component of fats) and transform them—through a series of intricate biochemical processes known as oxidation—into carbon dioxide, water, and energy for the body.

During the process of oxidation, free radicals are created. A free radical is an unpaired electron. Electrons are naturally paired together; and when one goes missing, the result is an unbalanced, electrically charged molecule that goes around looking for an electron to balance itself and will steal one from a protein, a fatty acid, or genetic material, creating more free radicals.

Oxidation is entropy—disorder—at work. During its brief life span of just a few thousandths of a second, a free radical can do considerable damage: splitting molecules in half, chipping pieces off them, and creating garbage that the body then has to get rid of.

Free radicals attack cell membranes, artery walls, DNA, collagen, and elastin. They are probably the most potent of the age-accelerating factors.

Doctors believe that free-radical damage plays a significant role in virtually every chronic, age-associated disease known today, including cancer, heart disease, Alzheimer's, arthritis, and diabetes.

This isn't a dramatic, shoot-'em-up kind of damage but a more subtle damage at the molecular level that accumulates over a lifetime. And free radicals are not all bad. They are necessary for immune system functioning, sending impulses through your nerves, making hormones, and contracting and relaxing muscles.

Each cell has an antioxidant system that quenches free radicals by donating electrons to them, a process called reduction. Most antioxidants, however, become free radicals themselves when they reduce other free radicals. Taking a broad spectrum of antioxidants allows each antioxidant to reduce others as it is oxidized.

Many of the foods we eat contain antioxidants—notably vitamins E and C, beta-carotene, and bioflavonoids—but the body also makes antioxidants, including glutathione, alpha lipoic acid, and coenzyme Q10. As we age, the body's production of these antioxidants decreases, so supplementing with antioxidant nutrients to help control free-radical damage makes excellent sense. One of the best supplements I have ever used is a combination of vitamin E and coenzyme Q10. More on this later.

Inflammation: A Valuable Immune Function Pushed Beyond Healthy Limits

Inflammation goes hand in hand with free radical production. Inflammation accelerates the production of free radicals.

Inflammation is an immune-system response that moves fluids (containing proteins and antibodies) and white blood cells (leukocytes) into areas of the body that have been injured. Inflammation assists in the repair of that injury. If you smack your head on something and it swells and turns red, you are experiencing inflammation. If you sprain your ankle or develop a skin infection, the redness and swelling you experience are inflammation in action. Fever is a whole-body state of inflammation.

But inflammation can also manifest more subtly. Inflammation within the walls of blood vessels can lead to heart attack or stroke. Modern research into heart disease—the cause of astronomical numbers of costly medical procedures and severe decreases in quality of life—reveals that an inflammatory process is at its root.

Chronic inflammation caused by bacteria or viruses is linked to some types of cancer. Repeated skin inflammations caused by sunburn throughout a person's life causes premature skin aging or, even worse, skin cancer.

In a weakened body, infection can cause inflammation to escalate to dangerously high levels. In the days before antibiotics, the body could only rely on its own ability to create inflammation to fend off microbial illnesses; sometimes that inflammatory fire would become so great that the resultant fever would kill the patient. Today, this rarely happens, but certain other kinds of chronic inflammations are more common than they were before antibiotics. Asthma, allergies, eczema, and psoriasis are all examples of chronic, low-grade inflammations. In more severe cases, uncontrolled inflammation can lead to autoimmune diseases such as lupus, rheumatoid arthritis, or multiple sclerosis. These ailments are very difficult to treat and are sometimes deadly.

Chronic psychological stress is yet another factor that worsens inflammation.

Glycation: If You Were a Broiled Chicken

If you'd like to gain awareness of what glycation is, take a look at a chicken browning in the oven. Notice that when you put a sweet glaze on that chicken, it browns faster and deeper. The proteins become hardened. If the chicken were still clucking, its body could no longer use these proteins, which would also be more prone to oxidation (more on this in a short while). This is glycation at work, and it happens in your body, too.

Glycation is the binding of glucose to protein. This process actually alters protein molecules, making them useless and causing damage to body tissues. Glycated proteins are particularly prone to oxidation: studies have found that they produce fifty times more free radicals than nonglycated proteins. High levels of oxidative stress further accelerate glycation.

Eating a lot of sugar and refined carbohydrates will take insulin levels on a roller-coaster ride, which will do more than make you fat: it will increase glycation reactions in your body. With glycation, the collagen (the main protein forming connective tissues) in your muscles and skin will get sticky and bunchy, causing your muscles to weaken. But you can, by implementing dramatic dietary changes, reverse this process. The time to start is now.

Large fluctuations in blood sugar and insulin levels accelerate the glycation process, causing type 2 diabetes. Obesity also appears to play a role. When we eat foods high in refined carbohydrates (such as grains with all the fiber and nutrients milled out) or sugar or even some natural whole foods like potatoes or bananas, the pancreas responds by producing a big rush of insulin. Eating these foods often results in chronically elevated insulin and blood sugar levels, maintaining a sugary "bath" for cells that promotes glycation. Over time, this kind of eating can lead to insulin resistance and hyperglycemia, both prediabetic conditions that often culminate in adult-onset diabetes.

Only one organ in the body needs sugar: the brain. Elsewhere in the body, where calories are adequate and many need storing, insulin's real job is to store them as fat. Your body is designed to respond to plentiful carbohydrates by storing fat away for the coming famine. When no famine comes, those fats hang around, with some released into the bloodstream as free fatty acids and triglycerides. The end result is increased buildup of fatty plaques in the heart's blood vessels.

THE DEADLY THREESOME

Oxidation, inflammation, and glycation are all age-accelerating factors and often interact. In the type 2 diabetic, for example, a combination of glycation, oxidation, and inflammation plus altered hormone levels, combine to accelerate aging exponentially. Thirty to 40 percent of randomly selected diabetic men suffer from low testosterone. They are likely to have low energy, low libido, and erection problems, and are at increased risk of heart, kidney, and blinding eye diseases. Being overweight, which most type 2 diabetics are, also lowers testosterone levels and increases inflammation throughout the body.

Let's take a closer look at the two most common diseases of aging, cardiovascular disease and type 2 diabetes, and how the big three both cause and spring from them. This is the kind of information that will cause you to pause when you're tempted to stray from your Age Optimization habits.

CARDIOVASCULAR DISEASE

Heart disease strikes many men and women during what should be the best years of their lives. It accounts for 44 percent of the annual deaths in the United States.

You might have no warning before heart disease strikes. You could have a heart attack or be diagnosed with coronary artery disease and end up in the hospital having bypass surgery. Believe me, this is something to avoid at all costs, even if you must give up french fries and hot fudge sundaes.

A heart attack is just one consequence of cardiovascular disease. Another is cholesterol-filled, inflamed plaque in the blood vessels. Plaque is more likely to form in the vessels that feed the heart muscle than anywhere else in the body because the heart muscles work so hard. Lying along the outer walls of the heart muscles, these vessels are in constant use and thus require a great deal of oxygen-rich blood. Shear stress is high in these arteries due to their torturous twists and turns along the heart's surface, enhancing the likelihood of damage to the inner lining of the vessels.

Plaque can be found elsewhere in the body, most often in the vessels of the brain, lower legs, and kidneys. Plaque formation begins with an injury to the muscular artery wall. The body attempts to repair the injury, depositing fatty substances (including cholesterol), calcium, and fibrin (a clotting agent in the blood). Then inflammation sets in, triggering immune factors that cause the plaque to grow and accelerating free-radical formation.

This inflammatory response spirals out of control when we eat foods that encourage inflammation. The plaque continues to grow, and a part can break off and float downstream to clog a narrower section of a blood vessel. Or the narrowed area where the plaque has developed might become occluded by a clot that migrated from elsewhere in the body. Another thing that can happen is that inflammation can cause a vessel to spasm, making the vessel clamp down and shut off blood flow through the occluded section. But no matter how the blood flow is stopped, the result is the same: the tissues downstream are deprived of oxygen.

If this happens in a heart vessel, a portion of the heart muscle can die. If it happens in the brain, this is called an occlusive stroke, and a portion of the brain can die. Doctors estimate that 25 percent of those who lose their memory or their ability to think clearly have experienced an undiagnosed mini-stroke. Additionally, the kidneys can fail, and nerves and muscles in the lower legs can waste away because of cardiovascular disease.

TYPE 2 DIABETES

According to Michael Roizen, MD, author of RealAge: Are You as Young as You Can Be? (Collins, 2001) and other books, diabetes ages you, on average, seven years. This means that a diabetic who is forty adds seven years to his or her real biological age.

Type 2 diabetes gives us a clear portrait of accelerated aging because it increases all of the big three—oxidation, inflammation, and glycation. Type 2 diabetics run a much higher risk of heart attack, stroke, and degenerative eye diseases. They are prone to kidney failure, gum disease, and circulatory deficiencies that can lead to gangrene and then amputation of toes, feet, even legs.

Insulin resistance, hyperglycemia, and type 2 diabetes accelerate the aging process significantly but can all be avoided with good eating, healthy weight, and exercise. Today, 90-95 percent of the 18.3 million people with diabetes in the United States have the type 2 variety, and these numbers are rising. More and more children are being affected by this disease, once known as "adult-onset diabetes."

A PROACTIVE APPROACH TO OPTIMIZING YOUR AGE

While the causes of aging are still not completely understood, modern medicine has developed some excellent diagnostic tests to detect signs and risk factors for cardiovascular disease and diabetes—the most common age-related diseases—long before life-threatening symptoms appear. These tests can determine whether you would benefit from supplemental hormones or nutrients and tell you what you need to know to stave off or at least postpone the changes that many think are inevitable parts of aging.

I recommend a complete panel of lab tests every six months. This allows you to catch any small deviation from health long before it becomes serious. This might sound excessive but consider the fact that traditional Chinese medicine (TCM)—a healing art that has been around for five thousand years—looks for even the slightest physical imbalances. TCM doctors study and train for years to diagnose and treat conditions long before they manifest as diseases. Modern medical testing enables us to do the same thing. If we properly interpret the test results and choose an appropriate course of action, we will be a lot better off in the long run. And in any case, lab work is a lot cheaper than major surgery.

In the appendices, you'll find the lab tests that I recommend, with information about how to interpret the results. You can bring this book to your doctor to help find out which of these tests you can get through him or her. Other tests you can order by mail, and these you can learn about in the resources section.

CHAPTER FOUR

Food Is A Drug: How To Eat Yourself Young

TODAY'S WESTERNERS HAVE overall become the fattest people in the history of the world. Fast foods and other junk foods, day after day, are adding millions of pounds to the Western population.

Modernity migrated people from farmland to the city. With the industrial and the information revolutions, untold blessings and advantages have come for some, but these revolutions have also brought problems. As farming became industrialized, food became abundant and relatively inexpensive; but that food was increasingly processed, sugared, injected with strange fats, artificially colored and flavored, wrapped in cellophane, boxed, or canned. The very nature of these foods encourages us to eat much more than needed—about 300-plus extra calories a day for men, about 160-plus calories for women.

A TV commercial for a fast-food burger restaurant depicts a young man standing in front of a supermarket aisle that is filled, floor to ceiling, with many brands of packaged, sliced bread. He looks overwhelmed and finally walks away, with a voice-over saying, "Without us, some guys would starve."

Some guys? How about most guys—and most girls? About 95 percent of the U.S. population would be hungry and helpless without adulterated, cellophane-wrapped, boxed, or canned foods from supermarket shelves.

In a world filled with processed, mouth-watering junk, the first step in resisting the daily temptation to eat foods that harm us is knowing exactly how they do so. This information will serve to expand your awareness, helping you to make better choices automatically. Once you know what that bowl of chips or piece of cake is doing to your body, you're far less likely to take a bite, much less overindulge.

THE KEY: FOOD LITERACY

The only way to create a truly healthful way of eating and stick with it is to become what I call food literate. A food-literate person understands what food does once it enters the body and how it affects his or her well-being and health in both the short and long term. A food-literate person will automatically avoid foods that will cause harm. She will know how to read labels and ask questions. Food literacy lets us see the interactions of the energies of air, water, food, and earth; and this understanding will inform the choices we make in the grocery store or restaurant.

Food literacy is the key to becoming aware of the effects of your diet on your body, mind, and soul. Food not only affects us at the cellular level but at the molecular and atomic levels. We rarely consider this when we chow down just to fill our stomachs, to lift our spirits, or to be social.

A lot of pseudoexperts have dubious theories about which foods are better than others. First-hand knowledge of what foods actually do in and to your body is what will benefit you the most. That way, your choices come from your own understanding, not from edicts coming from people who are more interested in making money with the next trendy diet plan than in actually being of service to you.

Publishers know they'll sell more copies of diet books that offer hard-and-fast formulas, specific recipes, and black-and-white dictums. The thing most diet books don't acknowledge is that every time you eat something, you are making a choice. If you are fat or have ailments related to poor eating, you are consistently making bad choices. This is not theory; it is fact.

Our critical relationships with food have been greatly affected by commerce and marketing. Brilliant marketers can't generate huge profits working for organic farmers, which means they can't pull down big salaries for themselves while helping you to make the best possible choices.

If you are not feeding your body with the foods that promote optimal weight and overall glowing good health, the first thing you need to do is acknowledge it and call it what it is. Until you do this, you will not be motivated to change your eating in the ways I will describe in this chapter. Simply acknowledge it: "I'm eating junk, and that is bad for my health." No excuses, no explanations. Stay in this moment and then look to the future. Ask yourself in a straightforward manner, "What do I do to change this?" Don't be one of those unfortunate individuals who requires a catastrophic health event to wake you up to a better way of eating.

Do you really need to lose weight? Isn't a little weight gain totally normal for a person who is past the blush of youth? Well, yes. Five pounds, maybe ten should not disrupt your health too much. You cannot expect to stay as hard-bodied as you were when you were twenty. But fifteen, twenty, thirty, fifty pounds? This kind of weight gain is not natural and will definitely damage your health.

Also keep in mind that you do not have to be overweight to be in poor health. Being thin does not give you a free pass to fill your body with garbage. Eating low-quality foods, even in moderation, will still age you prematurely, reduce your energy and spark, and give you heart disease, cancer, or some other chronic condition.

Anyone who tells you that you can lose weight and keep it off while eating as much as you want of the foods you love is blowing smoke. You also cannot go on a restrictive diet for a period of time and then go off that regimen without gaining the weight back. But know this: You can learn to enjoy new foods. And you can eat less of the foods you love and not suffer terribly. This isn't the end of the world. I promise you.

FOOD LITERACY FUNDAMENTALS

In recent years, I've performed an experiment on myself that never fails to yield the results I expect. I can gain and lose the same eight to ten pounds, in a matter of three or four days, simply by altering the relative amounts of protein, fat, and carbohydrate in my diet. You can do the same.

Standard refined, high-carbohydrate, high-sugar American fare sends insulin levels soaring and crashing, again and again. Eating this way is like training your body for the weight-gain event at the Olympics. People who eat the standard high-carbohydrate diet are creating abundant inflammation in their bodies. This inflammatory state damages your tissues and can be likened to a mild sunburn occurring throughout your body.

If you eat these kinds of foods and are overweight, the inflammation is even worse. Belly fat is particularly inflammatory; you'll find out why as you read on. The amount of C-reactive protein (C-RP) in your blood will give you a good idea of how much "inner sunburn" is going on in your body. You will find out more about the C-RP test in this chapter.

What takes hunger away is protein and fat. What promotes excellent overall health are vegetables, fruit, whole grains, nuts, seeds, and healthful fats from fish. Carbohydrates stoke the furnace—meaning that they cause insulin levels to rise and the body to quickly crave more carbohydrates as blood sugar drops. The simpler the carbohydrate (sugar is the simplest, and whole grains are the least simple), the higher the fire. If you get up in the morning and have a five-hundred-calorie white-flour bagel with low-fat spread, you're going to be ready for a five-course meal by 10:00 a.m.—or, at the very least, another generous helping of refined carbohydrates.

THE CURRENT STATE OF UNHEALTHY WEIGHT

Westerners generally underestimate their level of fatness. Since 2000, worldwide, there has been a marked increase in obesity even in third-world countries. Current estimates suggest that 250 million adults worldwide are overweight (body mass index of 30-35), with many of them being obese (BMI of 40 or more). About 127 million of these people are Americans—that's 64.5 percent of our adult population, overweight or obese.

Are You Overweight or Obese?

Here is the formula for calculating your body mass index (BMI):

BMI = weight in pounds/height in inches squared x 703

For example, if you are five feet, seven inches tall and weigh 205 pounds, you would divide 205 by 67 inches squared (4,489). That yields .0457. Then multiply that number by 703, which gives you a BMI of 32.1—which makes you overweight but not obese.

BMI calculators, where you enter your weight and height and your BMI is quickly calculated, can be found on the Internet.

A recent study by health economist Roland Sturm of the Rand Corporation showed that the number of Americans who weigh one hundred pounds or more over their ideal weight has quadrupled since 1986. In the mid-1980s, one in two hundred adults could be classified as extremely obese (one-hundred-plus pounds overweight), where today, one in fifty falls in this category.

How has this obesity epidemic happened? It's fundamentally not so much an epidemic of obesity as much as an epidemic of lack of awareness. Only a serious lack of awareness can allow a person to balloon to thirty, fifty, or one hundred to two hundred pounds overweight. Even those with a degree of awareness sometimes feel the need to indulge themselves in the momentary bliss of a "sinful" food. They might crave a piece of cake or high-calorie coffee drink with whipped cream on top. "Why not?" they might think. "I've worked so hard today. I deserve this!" Once this starts to happen every day, those calories add up! As you become more food literate, you will understand completely "why not," and you'll begin to seek pleasure elsewhere.

Of course, it's okay to occasionally have a small indulgence . . . a few french fries or a morsel of chocolate. Make sure these foods are made with unsaturated fat. Don't binge and make sure it's occasional and done with awareness, not habitual or unconscious. You might decide that Saturdays and Tuesdays are your days for having a little treat and mindfully indulge on those days while abstaining on others.

We can conceive of this so-called obesity epidemic in another way, as an epidemic of unhappiness—an epidemic lack of self-love, of a feeling of energy and excitement . . . so people try to find it in something quick, like sweet food. We all know how that internal monologue goes: Oooh,

I think it's time for a treat . . . I'm going to go to the bakery aisle and get myself something delicious! That thrill might not be monumental, but on the average day, it can brighten things up considerably. But keep in mind that this avenue to brief bliss is going to put pounds on your frame and adversely affect your health.

Obesity and overweight are often treated as merely cosmetic issues. While I think that they need to be addressed as health issues first and foremost, the desire to look good can serve as a great motivator. Most people enjoy physical beauty, admire it in others, and would like to be more beautiful themselves. When their bodies are in good shape, they feel energized.

Your inner life can even improve as a result of looking better: you may feel happier and more confident. Looking good is an easy way to get people to look at you and give you their energy.

You cannot get there by eating foods that give you momentary pleasure but don't nourish you. Sugar, salt, and saturated fats can taste terrific but will sooner or later undermine your health. That much, you can count on. Once you see how the typical modern Western way of eating stresses your cells out, once you really see what you are doing to your body when you eat a doughnut or a piece of fatty cured meat, that awareness will inform and ultimately change your behavior. But you must truly see it and keep it in your awareness, despite the discomfort you will probably experience.

TEMPTATION

Overweight and obesity are the product of ongoing errors in judgment and behavior, usually from eating too much of the wrong foods time after time after time. For you to prevail over obesity, you must remain focused on the choices you make at each and every meal, with each and every snack.

As you move into this new awareness and a better way of eating, you can expect temptations and lapses. Don't become discouraged. Even Jesus and Buddha succumbed to temptation. See the little devils of temptation and lapsing as what they truly are: teachers.

Don't think, "I am so weak, how could I screw up like this, I'll never lose this weight!" Think instead, "I made a poor choice today, I didn't treat my body as well as I should have, and I'm going to make a better choice right now." Each time you eat, you have an opportunity to make a choice that is nourishing and life-giving. What a gift!

Do you overindulge habitually? Do you have trouble resisting temptation? Then get the bad stuff out of your refrigerator, your house, and your life. Don't tempt yourself.

EATING WELL IS ABOUT MORE THAN LOSING WEIGHT

All around us we can see the effects of American obesity. The Federal Aviation Administration has mandated that airlines add ten pounds to approved passenger weights. Airline, theater, and stadium seats have been widened to accommodate American passengers, moviegoers, and sports fans.

In the 1950s, calipers were developed for the measurement of body fat. Today, 25 percent of women in their fifties are too fat to be measured with this instrument. Clothes-sizing standards have been changed so that a woman who wore a size 14 in the 1940s is now a size 10. Hypodermic needles are now longer too because of all the fat they have to penetrate before they can draw blood from the average patient's bloodstream or administer a drug.

Being overweight or obese will have devastating effects on your health, and the more extra pounds you carry, the worse your health will be. Obesity both leads to and worsens the following conditions:

- Arthritis
- Asthma
- Breast, uterine, colon, and prostate cancers
- Breastfeeding failure
- Chronic lower-back pain
- Cor pulmonale (a type of heart failure)
- Coronary artery disease, heart attack, stroke
- Gallstones

- Gastroesophageal reflux disease (GERD), which can lead to esophageal ulceration and perhaps even asthma
- Hernia
- Herniated vertebral discs (where the fluid-filled discs between the vertebrae are damaged and leak, causing inflammation and often excruciating back pain)
- High LDL cholesterol
- High triglycerides
- Hypertension
- Increased inflammation
- Infertility, pregnancy complications, gestational diabetes
- Menstrual disorders
- Obesity hypoventilation syndrome (in which breathing is depressed due to changes in central nervous system functioning)
- Obstructive sleep apnea (where the sufferer's excess weight causes airway blockage, resulting in daytime drowsiness and loud snoring and long pauses in breathing during the night)
- Pulmonary hypertension (high blood pressure in the blood vessels of the lungs)
- Recurrent heartburn
- Skin disorders related to diabetes and hygiene problems
- Type 2 diabetes
- Unwanted hair growth in women
- Urinary incontinence and frequent urinary tract infections
- Thin people can have these problems too although they are much more characteristic of fat people. Ultimately, very few people who are truly aware of what they eat and how it affects their bodies suffer from these conditions.

A thin person doesn't need ice cream sundaes, greasy tortilla chips, or processed meats any more than a fat person does. When the foods eaten are the right foods, eaten with awareness, the appetite takes care of itself.

THE ROLE OF HABIT

When I check a patient's reflexes, I often do something that illustrates the role of habit in making lifestyle choices. I tap the knee with my reflex hammer twice, and the knee jerks twice. Then, I pretend I am going to tap a third time, stopping short, and the patient's knee jerks anyway.

Most of us, when we sit down to eat, habitually shovel food into our mouths because we are used to being in a hurry to get to the next thing we believe we must do. And when something tastes delicious, many of us eat as much of it as we can get. Slick advertising campaigns for unhealthy foods are so effective that by the time we get around to a meal, we don't remember the commercials and have no idea why we feel the urge to eat generous helpings of that food or guzzle down that drink—we just know that we want to!

Awareness can break these habits. Specifically, the awareness of how food gives each and every cell in our bodies, each tissue, and every organ the fuel and other nutrients they require to work smoothly in concert.

HOW FOOD AFFECTS YOUR BODY AND MIND

Food impacts your physiology in many ways, with its main effects falling into two categories:

1. Its effects on the crucial hormones insulin and glucagon (GLUE-kuh-gon), which regulate the amount of glucose (simple sugar) in your bloodstream, how much of it is stored as fat, and the passage of fuel into individual cells, where it is transformed into energy
2. Its effects on the hormone-like biochemicals called eicosanoids (eye-KAH-suh-noyds), which play many roles in regulating inflammation, blood circulation, and immune function

Lipid biochemist Barry Sears was the first to apply the concept of food as drug. This chapter would never have been written, and a great many people would probably still be following the ridiculous advice to eat mostly carbohydrates, without the benefit of his work. The ideas in this section also glean a great deal from the work of Dr. Robert Atkins, who bravely told the world that carbohydrates, not protein and fat, are what make us fat.

The world-famous "Zone" plan developed by Dr. Sears told readers to eat a precise ratio of protein to carbohydrate to fat to control insulin and eicosanoid levels. Once this plan had been implemented, the patient was said to be "in the Zone," where he or she would feel better, look better, and live longer. Dr. Sears's research and books have helped to create literacy about controlling eicosanoids and insulin to control weight and energy levels and prevent disease. Dr. Sears's first book came out in the early 1990s after the eicosanoids had been acknowledged and studied by the scientific community for almost one hundred years.

Unfortunately, mainstream medicine has not yet completely recognized the importance of the eicosanoids and insulin in preventing aging and chronic diseases. Although a recent search for eicosanoid in the National Library of Medicine's database returned 98,247 hits—that's 98,247 different research studies on eicosanoids published in peer-reviewed journals—if you go ask your doctor for help in controlling your eicosanoids, she might just give you a blank stare.

Change takes time. Remember Ignaz Semmelweis, the physician who first suggested that delivery-room doctors should wash their hands between patients. Semmelweis was lambasted for his theories that doctors' hands were spreading childbed fever (puerperal sepsis), a disease that killed many women in maternity wards in those days. Doctors were enraged at the idea that their hands could transmit deadly sepsis. Tragically, many years passed before Semmelweis's ideas were acknowledged and put into widespread practice. Someday the medical community will be saying the same thing about Sears, eicosanoids and insulin, and their links to deadly age-related diseases.

The Atkins diet can quickly remove pounds from the body. It is all about controlling insulin by strictly limiting carbohydrates but does not even address eicosanoids. An optimal diet has to consider both.

The brilliant Zone plan turned a lot of people off because it was complicated and rigid, and required precise computation of portion sizes and seemingly odd food combinations. Let's pare down the concepts of using food to control eicosanoids and insulin control so that you can build your food literacy.

INFLAMMATION: THE COMMON DENOMINATOR

Levels of insulin, glucagon, and eicosanoids all powerfully influence the variable that is the most important predictor of how long you will live and how you will look when you die: inflammation.

A food is like a drug in that it also influences our bodies' production of these biochemicals, which in turn control inflammation, decay, aging, and death.

Inflammation is an immune process that is crucial for survival. When you get an infection, your body creates a localized inflammation—redness, heat, swelling, and pain—due to the presence of immune cells that have migrated to the infected area to kill the invading germs and repair the tissue damage. Before antibiotics, people often died from the inflammation that accompanied infectious diseases: The "fire" that cleansed the body ended up burning the "house" down.

Today, we enjoy protection from all but the most virulent infectious diseases; but inflammation still burns inside our bodies, chronically and silently. I like to describe it as a sort of "inner sunburn" that lingers on, slowly "cooking" the tissues and aging them prematurely. When we take steps to cool this inner heat, we restore our tissues and slow aging. In a sense, this is like getting younger. We get stronger too. And we control inflammation by controlling eicosanoid and insulin levels with diet.

If you don't control your eicosanoids, your insulin, and your inflammation, you are (forgive me) screwed. You will experience pain and be unhappy. Indeed, chronic inflammation can make your life a living hell for decades before you finally kick the bucket.

Belly Fat and Your Heart

Glance down at your middle. Are you holding a big shelf of belly fat in your lap? Or just a little tummy you wish you could get rid of? Here's some motivation to eradicate that extra abdominal baggage.

Belly fat is a storage depot for arachidonic acid (AA), which is the building block for all the inflammatory eicosanoids. More metabolically active than hip or thigh fat, belly fat cranks out AA and other inflammatory substances, causing a cascade of inflammation throughout the body.

It has long been known that belly fat is more of a heart disease risk factor than fat in the thighs, hips, or rear end. This is why.

Time to get out the tape measure. Measure your waist at the level of your belly button. If you're male and your waist is thirty-six inches or more, your risk of disease is elevated. Better get moving. If you're a woman, a waist of thirty-one inches or larger is cause for increased focus on your diet and workout programs.

With increasing awareness of the hazards of chronic inflammation, the gold standard for testing full-body inflammation—C-reactive protein testing—is becoming more available. Ask your doctor to administer this test. Your C-RP levels should ideally be close to zero. If they aren't, make the changes I suggest and take the test again.

Fasting insulin testing has long been standard for the forty-and-over physical exam. Have this test regularly, anytime you go in for a physical, to make sure your insulin levels and responses fall in the safe zone.

A more recently developed test, the silent inflammation profile (SIP), offers a more high-tech measurement of inflammation that looks at the ratio of AA (arachidonic acid) to EPA (eicosapentaenoic acid). This test is still not commonly performed; Barry Sears, in his terrific book The Anti-Inflammation Zone, recommends contacting Nutrasource Diagnostics in Canada for an SIP.

Excessive and chronic inflammation will cause problems. Some people's bodies are more prone to these types of inflammations because of their genes. These are the individuals who develop autoimmune disease, allergies, asthma, eczema, and other chronic inflammatory conditions. Inflammation has been implicated as a major cause of Alzheimer's disease, chronic pain, and arthritis. Strong evidence affirms the link between chronic inflammation and heart disease. People vulnerable to these diseases can decrease their vulnerability with an anti-inflammatory diet—a diet that fosters the production of beneficial eicosanoids and keeps insulin and blood sugar low.

Inflammation is the most potent age-accelerator around. Diabetics know this firsthand. Diabetes leads to chronically high insulin and blood sugar levels, which keep the body in a constant state of inflammation. Inflammation accelerates tissue aging, hampers tissue repair, and accelerates the production of free radicals.

Oxidation and inflammation go hand in hand. Chronically high insulin levels worsen both oxidation and inflammation by causing pro-inflammatory changes in eicosanoid balance, resulting in a general state of physical decay.

THE EICOSANOIDS: SELF-HEALERS

Eicosanoid is a word derived from eicos, the Greek word for the number 20 because all eicosanoids are derived from essential fatty acids that are twenty carbons long. Eicosanoids are made in every cell and play a major role in nearly every physiological function.

Some sources, including Dr. Sears's books, use the terms eicosanoids and hormones interchangeably, confusing two distinct biochemicals. Most hormones—including testosterone, estrogen, progesterone, cortisol, DHEA, and growth hormone—are endocrine secretions, meaning they pass directly from the gland where they're made and into the circulatory system. They act globally, on both nearby and distant tissues. Eicosanoids, on the other hand, are exocrine and act locally on the cell where they are made or on adjacent cells. Eicosanoids act fast, then dissipate within seconds of their manufacture.

Hormones are not directly affected by food choices, but eicosanoids—both their production and activity—are directly and dramatically influenced by the food one chooses to eat.

Eicosanoids are ancient. They were the first hormones, produced by living organisms at least 500 million years ago. Every single one of the 60 trillion (or more) cells in the human body makes eicosanoids. Eicosanoids are produced within seconds, do their work, then dissolve. Their fleeting nature makes them difficult to study, but this hasn't stopped the scientific community from trying. More than one hundred types of eicosanoids have been discovered so far.

Eicosanoids are built from fatty acids, which are the building blocks of fat in the foods we eat. To understand how eicosanoids work, you have to understand the basics about fats.

FATS AND FATTY ACIDS

All fats (including solid fats like butter and lard) and oils (like olive and canola) are built from fatty acids. Fatty acids range in length from four carbons (butyric acid) to twenty-four carbons (nisinic acid, a healthful omega-3 fatty acid). A saturated fat such as butter or lard remains solid at room temperature; a partly saturated fat such as chicken fat or olive oil is liquid at room temperature and solid when refrigerated; and a highly unsaturated fat, like fish oil or flax seed oil, is always liquid. All are strings of carbon molecules.

When three fatty acids and a "backbone" of a sugar called glycerol group together, they form triglycerides. Triglycerides float through your bloodstream trying to find (1) fat cells to be stored in, or (2) cells where they can be "burned" to release energy. When the fat you eat is absorbed by your body, the triglycerides it contains are broken down into glycerol and fatty acids. Once in the bloodstream, the triglyceride components re-form to triglycerides and transport fat in your body.

Fatty acids can also attach to cholesterol, which is one of a family of compounds called alcohols. Cholesterol is neither a fat nor a fatty acid, and although it occurs in many of the same foods as fats and fatty acids, it plays a different role in the body.

The amount of fatty acid in a cut of meat (or in the animal's milk) varies depending on what that animal ate. If it's a cow that grazed on fresh green grass, its flesh is going to have a more healthful fatty acid composition than if it was fed the usual factory farming diet. The fatty acid in a piece of fish will be more healthful if the fish ate wild, natural, omega-3–rich algae or krill than if it subsisted on grain-based food in a fish farm.

Fatty acids, like carbohydrates, are also used to make energy within cells. You might be surprised to learn that the human brain is composed of 60 percent fat. Fatty acids also function in making cell membranes, providing needed eicosanoids for new cells being created by the body. Many fatty acids can be made from other fatty acids within the body, and these are called "nonessential." Two vital classes of fatty acids are the omega-3s and the omega-6s. The most common saturated fatty acid, arachidonic acid, for example, is an omega-6.

Each of these types of fatty acids—omega-3 and omega-6—produces a distinct type of eicosanoid. This is why the fatty acid composition of the foods you eat directly affects your day-to-day state of wellness or ill health.

Enzymes convert omega-6s and omega-3s into eicosanoids, with the omega-6s being made into "bad" eicosanoids and the omega-3s becoming "good" eicosanoids. Most Westerners ingest too much omega-6—that is, too many short-chain, saturated and trans fats—and too few long-chain omega-3 fats.

Many believe that the evolution of the highly intelligent brain of modern humans was at least partly due to the eating of fish and other sea creatures containing omega-3 fatty acids. This began about one hundred fifty thousand years ago and is thought to have accelerated the development of the forebrain in particular, the part of the brain that enables us to think and reason.

In Paleolithic times, the ratio of omega-6 to omega-3 fats in the typical day-to-day diet was about 1:1, but today it's at least 10:1. Optimal eicosanoid balance can be restored by increasing omega-3s and reducing omega-6s in the diet.

"GOOD" AND "BAD" EICOSANOIDS

I put "bad" and "good" in quotation marks because all the eicosanoids perform necessary functions. The problem begins when inflammatory, constricting, blood pressure—raising eicosanoids are overproduced and those that are anti-inflammatory, opening, and blood pressure—lowering are underproduced. And this is the case in the bodies of the vast majority of people who consume a standard Western diet.

Eicosanoids affect

- *mood, memory, and cognitive functioning.* Lack of omega-3 fats and the eicosanoids they are made into have been linked to bipolar disorder, mood swings, postpartum depression, Alzheimer's disease, and poor memory. Babies who are breast-fed get more omega-3 fats than formula-fed babies, and they perform better on intelligence and vision tests and are less likely to have learning disabilities or behavioral problems later on. Omega-3 fats are now commonly added to baby formulas.
- *blood pressure.* The balance of fatty acids and eicosanoids greatly affects the contractility of the muscular walls of the arteries. When bad eicosanoids prevail, blood vessel walls constrict, and blood pressure rises. Reestablishing the balance of good and bad enables blood vessel walls to relax and open, lowering blood pressure and increasing blood flow.
- *thrombosis.* This is the medical term for a blood clot. Eicosanoids affect clot formation in the bloodstream, with bad eicosanoids increasing clotting, especially in the vessels of the brain, heart, legs, and lungs.
- *skin health.* When bad eicosanoids overwhelm good, skin can become too dry (flaky and itchy) or too oily (leading to acne). Proper fatty acid balance promotes healthy, smooth, supple skin.
- *smooth-muscle tension.* Smooth-muscle tissue lines the blood vessels and the intestines. Eicosanoid imbalance creates excessive muscle tension throughout the body.
- *immune function.* The "bad" eicosanoids have a noble purpose: enhancing immune system response. They increase the number of immune cell "troops" that target, kill, and digest pathogens and dead tissue. When these eicosanoids are out of balance with the good ones, however, the immune response overresponds and lingers, doing harm along with good.

MODULATING EICOSANOIDS WITH DIET

Less omega-6, more omega-3: this is your formula for good eicosanoid balance. The best sources of omega-3 fats are fish that come from deep, cold waters.

Wild fish get their omega-3s from algae. Farm-raised fish are fed largely the fish version of the standard American diet. They live in more polluted waters than their wild brethren. And so wild-caught fish—especially salmon—are your best source of omega-3s. Omega-6s are most abundant in processed foods, especially those containing soybean oil, corn oil, safflower oil, sunflower oil, and cottonseed oil.

Because of the high level of mercury contamination of the world's oceans and because of the very real risk that overfishing poses to ocean ecosystems, I cannot advise you to eat fish more than three times a week. Eat salmon when you eat fish, if possible, because it's less contaminated than any other commonly consumed fish. Completely avoid mackerel, tilefish, shark, albacore tuna, and swordfish.

Even that mainstay of the American meal tuna is questionable at this point. If you eat canned tuna, eat "chunk light" tuna, which has less mercury contamination than albacore; and eat it only once a week. Mercury is a heavy metal, and like other heavy metals, exposure to it increases the risk of heart disease and Alzheimer's disease. It's a potent neurotoxin that kills brain cells, and it promotes oxidation and inflammation in both the brain and blood vessels.

I advise everyone to take omega-3 fatty acid supplements, even if they eat fish. I'll explain how to choose the best possible omega-3 supplement and how much to take later on.

As you increase the omega-3 fats in your food and decrease the omega-6 fats, also reduce your intake of simple sugars and refined flour. Eating a lot of simple carbohydrates like flour and sugar will alter enzyme activity so that your cells begin to crank out more bad eicosanoids even if you increase your intake of omega-3s and decrease your omega-6s.

What about other sources of omega-3 fats? Flaxseeds, traditionally known as linseeds, are rich in an omega-3 fatty acid called alpha linolenic acid (ALA). Oatmeal, canola oil, pumpkin seeds, walnuts, and the medicinal oils from blackcurrant seeds also contain ALA, although only a fraction of the amount found in flax. Flax oil is widely touted as the ideal omega-3 supplement for those who don't want to eat fish.

Unlike DHA and EPA, the ALA molecule is a short-chain omega-3. To be made into good eicosanoids, ALA molecules must be transformed into long-chain omega-3s. Some people's bodies are better at making this conversion than others. Flaxseeds, oatmeal, and walnuts are good foods; but don't rely on them to give you the omega-3 fats you require. Ground flaxseeds are great for the digestive system; they nourish the friendly bacteria in the colon, which promote healthy elimination and help us to absorb nutrients from the foods we eat.

SATURATED FAT: EAT IN MODERATION

Saturated fats are solid at room temperature and are found in most animal foods, including beef, poultry, eggs, butter, and coconut and palm kernel oils. I recommend that you avoid solid fats whenever possible. Many studies have shown that saturated fats cause cholesterol to rise, with other research showing that a meal rich in saturated fat causes blood vessels to constrict in the hours that follow.

When you can, use monounsaturated oils instead—olive, canola, and peanut oils. For baking, if a solid oil is required, don't use margarine or shortening. Use coconut oil or butter instead and eat whatever you are making in moderation. When you prepare a fried dish, fry at a lower temperature and use a monounsaturated fat like canola, peanut, or olive oil.

If you want a buttery flavor on your vegetables, try Smart Choice or other spread made with a healthful combination of oils. (Some of these oil combinations have been found to lower cholesterol.) Having a couple of eggs in the morning is fine although I recommend that you discard at least one of the yolks. When you consume meats, eat no more than five or six ounces at a time.

A cup of plain, organic, low-fat yogurt is a good choice for a snack. Toss some frozen blueberries in for an ice cream-like treat or add other low-glycemic fresh fruit.

Don't eat huge portions of meat, dairy, or poultry. Chew foods longer than you think you need to until they are liquid in your mouth. You will find that your appetite is satisfied sooner, and you will have less digestive discomfort.

Anytime you eat saturated fats, take a gram (1000 milligrams) of omega-3s along with them. I carry a few in my pocket to take with each meal. Keep in mind that while supplemental vitamins and minerals are helpful in a case like this, they still won't solve your inflammation problems. Only careful manipulation of the exocrine hormones (eicosanoids) can rein in chronic slow-burning inflammation.

> **Not All Olive Oils Are Created Equal**
>
> Research on the Mediterranean diet and on olive oil, an important ingredient of that diet, strongly suggest that this oil protects against heart disease, stroke, cancer, and other ills linked to the overconsumption of wrong kinds of oils.
>
> Olive oil is classified as an omega-9 oil. As far as eicosanoid production goes, it is neutral. Olive oil that is imported, extra-virgin, and cold-pressed is the highest-quality grade of olive oil. It is minimally processed and can be as delicious as a glass of fine wine. It is rich in a polyphenol called hydroxytyrosol, which is one of our most potent antioxidant substances.
>
> Many supermarket olive oils are adulterated with other oils, or are of inferior quality. I get my olive oil from Olio2go, a company in Fairfax, Virginia that imports Italy's best olive oils. You can order from the company's Web site, www.olio2go.com, or peruse your market for extra-virgin oils made overseas.

AVOID TRANS FATS

Hydrogenation is a process that improves the shelf life of polyunsaturated oils, which tend to spoil quickly. Hydrogenated oils are cheaper to make than saturated or monounsaturated oils (such as olive, canola, and peanut) but aren't good for baking or frying because they are liquid and spoil easily.

A recent series of studies have shown that margarine and other foods rich in trans fats are worse for the health of the circulatory system than any other fat. Trans fats increase free-radical production, adversely affect cholesterol balance, and increase heart disease risk. Studies have shown that trans fat consumption increases inflammation and lowers "good" HDL and raises "bad" LDL, while increasing levels of lipoprotein(a), a protein known to increase heart attack risk.

Restaurants fry in this kind of oil; and most commercially available chips, crackers, fried foods, snack foods, and baked goods also contain them. As of this writing, labeling laws that require information about trans fat content have been passed, and many processed food makers are phasing out these bad fats. In California, restaurants have to notify patrons if they use trans fats; they have been banned in New York City restaurants.

The research on trans fats shows clearly that they are harmful in even small quantities and should be avoided entirely. And note that a product label declaring zero trans fats doesn't mean it actually contains none; anything under half a gram per serving can be called zero on the label. If the item contains any hydrogenated or partially hydrogenated vegetable oil, put it back on the grocery store shelf and find something else to eat.

CHOLESTEROL: HOW MUCH IS TOO MUCH?

Cholesterol is a type of fat found in all cell membranes. When we eat eggs, dairy products, or meats, we are eating cholesterol. Most of the cholesterol in your body right now, however—80 percent—was made in your liver. This is the kind of cholesterol affected by statin drugs like Lipitor. The other 20 percent of the cholesterol in your body came from your diet. When you eat foods high in cholesterol, your liver makes less.

In the United States, 102.3 million people have cholesterol counts of 200 mg/dL (milligrams per deciliter) or higher, and 41.3 million have 240 mg/dL or higher. Around half of white American men have an LDL (the "bad" kind of cholesterol) of 130 or greater; around 40 percent of American women do too, as do 46 percent of black men and 43 percent of Hispanic men. These numbers are too high. Cholesterol this high increases risk of heart attacks and strokes.

What causes cholesterol to rise too high? Cholesterol in your food does have some influence, but the bulk of the research points to saturated fats having a stronger influence on cholesterol levels. A high intake of sugars or other refined carbohydrates will also cause cholesterol to rise.

To protect yourself against cardiovascular disease, keep your total cholesterol as low as possible. Optimal total cholesterol is 140 or below, with an HDL of at least 40. Keep your LDL at around 60 or 70 if you can. As noted earlier, HDL is the good cholesterol that cleans the bad LDL from the artery walls.

"My total cholesterol is 200, and my doctor said that was just fine," you might say. Total cholesterol of 150 and HDL of 35 are accepted by the medical mainstream, but these numbers are not optimal. The optimization approach swoops right by the mediocrity and low standards of the health and medical establishment and goes for the absolute pinnacle of health and well-being. The preponderance of scientific evidence today suggests that the lower the LDL and the higher the HDL, the better your health, and I very much endorse this idea with my patients.

A newer test, the VAP (vertical auto profile) test, measures HDL, LDL, triglycerides, and total cholesterol, just like the older tests; but it also measures several subclasses of cholesterol. Together, all these measurements enable your doctor to much more accurately predict your risk of cardiovascular disease. If you can get this test, do so.

I put patients who have a hard time controlling their cholesterol on statin drugs. These drugs are remarkable, with research showing that they might have anti-inflammatory effects strong enough to protect against Alzheimer's disease.

If you take statin drugs, please be sure to take the supplement called coenzyme Q10 (coQ10). Statins deplete coQ10, a nutrient very important for heart health. Periodic liver testing is also a must for those who take statins.

New markers for heart disease risk have been discovered in recent years. The level of C-reactive protein (a marker of inflammation) could prove to be an important predictor of coronary artery disease, fully as important as cholesterol. Controlling eicosanoids with the right food choices, losing weight, and taking high-dose fish oil supplements will maintain suitable C-reactive protein levels for most people.

Brushing and Flossing for the Health of Your Heart

Gum disease and heart attacks often occur in the same people. Why? Because having gingivitis or periodontal disease somehow increases your risk of developing plaque along the walls of the heart's arteries. This probably reflects the body's heightened and chronic state of inflammation, exacerbated by pathogenic bacteria irritating the gums.

Proper care and feeding of the gums are important in keeping inflammation at bay throughout the body. Brush after eating and floss once or twice a day. Replace your toothbrush every month or two and be sure to clean the brush well between uses.

If you have periodontal disease—gums that are swollen and bleed easily—have it treated by a dentist and take steps to keep the disease from recurring.

THE WHITER THE SUGAR, THE QUICKER YOU DIE: INSULIN AND GLUCAGON, REVISITED

Now you know that fats are not the bad guys, and they are not responsible for making two-thirds of Americans fat. They are not solely responsible for the epidemic of chronic disease either. What is making us so fat and so sick? Too many carbohydrates.

Unhealthy carbohydrates—sugar, white flour—are not in and of themselves bad, but they do raise insulin and lower glucagon. This means that they inflame your body, clog up your system, and age you. They clog up your circulatory system and enhance inflammation.

Carbohydrates (also known as starches) are molecules that contain carbon, hydrogen, and oxygen bound together in a ring shape. One group of carbohydrates is the simple sugars: the monosaccharides, which include glucose, fructose, and galactose, all carbohydrates made up of a single "ring"; and the disaccharides, composed of two monosaccharides bound together. The common disaccharide sucrose, or white table sugar, is composed of one fructose and one glucose molecule.

In nature, most carbohydrates exist as polysaccharides—groupings of ten or more carbohydrate rings bound together. When digested, polysaccharides are broken down into simple sugars and passed into the bloodstream.

How about those carbohydrates that consist of simple sugars bound together? These are the oligosaccharides. Oligosaccharides are not broken down during digestion but move intact into the lower gastrointestinal tract, where they feed the friendly bacteria that live there.

Fiber is a form of carbohydrate that the digestive juices cannot break down, at least not completely. Foods rich in fiber are digested more slowly than foods lacking fiber.

We need some carbs, yes, but we need to choose the right kind of carbs. Carbohydrates don't hurt us if we eat them in moderation. As is the case with fats, carbohydrates come in beneficial and not-so-beneficial forms. The many types of carbs exert strong effects on the body. Our bodies require energy from carbohydrates, and our brains prefer carbohydrate energy over that of the slower-burning fats.

When you take a bunch of wheat berries, strip off their husks, remove their germ, extract their oils, and grind them up into flour, you are removing fats, fiber, and nutrients; and you're left with little more than sugar. Processed food manufacturers sometimes put back some of the nutrition they remove by adding B vitamins and fiber. But a cupful of white flour is about as far from a handful of wheat berries as you can get without alchemical powers. Processing takes all the life out of food, all its vibrational energy.

When you take kernels of corn and transform them into high-fructose corn syrup, you have a substance that sends the taste buds into overdrive while providing next to no nutritional value. It's pure energy, pure empty calories.

Refined carbohydrates are much more calorically dense than complex carbohydrates. You can easily eat a whole day's worth of calories in the form of a crusty French baguette with butter before you even start on your entrée. Every day a lot of people drink a giant-sized soda, which contains more than 500 calories of sugar in the form of high-fructose corn syrup, without a second thought. Try downing 500 calories' worth of brown rice, fatty fish, or broccoli without awareness. Even if you did, the health risks would be minimal!

"Good" complex carbohydrates such as wheat berries, corn, oats, and brown rice are metabolized more slowly than their refined counterparts. The digestive tract must first break down the carbohydrates' fiber and proteins before they can enter the bloodstream as glucose, the simplest form of sugar. Highly refined carbohydrates, conversely, are more rapidly digested and pass quickly into the bloodstream. Blood sugar shoots way up.

Then the pancreas, a small organ located behind the stomach that monitors your blood sugar level, responds by producing more insulin. Insulin lowers your blood sugar by moving glucose into the cells to be used for energy, or into fat cells or muscle where it is stored for future use. The more refined the carbohydrate, the more abrupt the insulin response, and the more rapidly blood sugar drops after you ingest it. That's the "blood sugar crash" that gives you the shakes, makes you feel weak and dizzy, and causes you to crave more fast-acting carbohydrates. Ingesting more carbs leads to another insulin spike, after which you crash again. It's a vicious cycle.

Chronically spiking insulin levels have many undesirable effects in the body, including

- wild swings in energy and mood;
- increasing levels of fats in the blood, like cholesterol and triglycerides, by promoting fatty-acid synthesis in the liver;
- inhibiting the breakdown of body fat, particularly in adipose tissue (that's medical-ese for belly rolls, rear end "dimples," and other

fat-storage depots), which leads your body to fuel its energy needs with carbohydrates stored in the liver;
- producing body fat; insulin promotes the transformation of carbohydrates into fat, which then gets stored away in fat cells;
- stimulating appetite for carbs, causing you to feel hungry for more of the same an hour after eating.

Years of this kind of yo-yoing of blood sugar and insulin, coupled with being overweight, leads to the development of a condition called insulin resistance. This is the first step toward type 2 diabetes. Insulin resistance is in essence an attempt by an overfed body to decrease the amount of carbohydrate energy that can pass into its cells. Blood sugars remain high because the body's cells can't accept any more glucose.

High blood sugar is enormously damaging to the walls of blood vessels. So is chronically high insulin, which results when the pancreas pumps too much of the stuff to try to force glucose into the cells, despite their resistance. This is why type 2 diabetes can lead to coronary artery disease, stroke, erectile dysfunction, and kidney failure. Each of these ailments just reflects clogged blood vessels—in the heart, brain, penis, and kidneys, respectively.

We don't need simple sugar. We don't need it at all. The only organ that requires it is the brain, and your body can make that sugar from complex carbohydrates—or even from fat, if it has to. We are supposed to be burning fat, not sugars. You're far better off eating an avocado or swallowing three tablespoons of olive oil than you are eating a piece of bread.

The hormone glucagon is Abel to insulin's Cain. It's the good guy when it comes to optimizing your body's use of fuel. Glucagon is made in the pancreas like insulin, but its actions are opposite to those of insulin. It increases with low blood sugar and decreases with high blood sugar. High insulin levels also suppress glucagon release. Glucagon stimulates the burning of fat for energy while insulin stimulates fat storage.

When you eat a food that is primarily protein, such as fish or poultry or a low-carbohydrate protein shake, your body responds by increasing glucagon production. Eating protein (along with plenty of vegetables and fruit) will help you to become slimmer and live longer. One of my favorite glucagon-boosting snacks is a glass of cold soy milk with a scoop of whey protein blended in.

If you consume refined carbohydrates along with your protein, your insulin response will overwhelm your glucagon response. Choose small amounts of nutrient-dense, complex carbohydrates with your protein. For example, instead of a cheeseburger on a fluffy white-flour bun, have some almond butter with a few whole-grain crackers, or apple with cheese, or baked tofu slices on a salad.

If you must have a food rich in refined carbs, first have a bit of protein with vegetables. Eating quick-burning carbohydrates with a high glycemic index (GI) along with protein and fat will actually suppress glucagon production, so take a half hour or hour between your balanced meal and your sweet indulgence.

CARBOHYDRATES AND THE BRAIN

Is there such a thing as carbohydrate addiction? Yes, but what's really going on is addiction to serotonin and beta-endorphin, two neurotransmitters that have calming and cheering effects. Levels of both of these neurotransmitters rise when you eat carbohydrates.

Alcohol addiction is known to run in families. Some contemporary studies have found a similar genetic pattern in carbohydrate addiction. A few researchers have even suggested they are one and the same. When carbohydrate addicts try to kick their habit, their experiences can be a lot like those of people addicted to alcohol and other substances, including withdrawal symptoms and emotional breakdowns. I mention this not to dissuade you from kicking your carb habit but to let you know what you might expect, and to steel yourself for that.

OPTIMAL EATING GUIDELINES, PART I: LOW-GLYCEMIC, ANTI-INFLAMMATORY

In my own clinical and personal experience, maintaining blood sugar and insulin at optimal levels is one of the most important things you can do to remain in a youthful state of good health. Accomplishing this will also keep inflammation at bay by promoting optimal eicosanoid balance. An enormous body of research supports me on this.

You do this by

- eating low on the glycemic index;
- avoiding omega-6-rich foods high in polyunsaturated vegetable fats (soybean, corn, sunflower, safflower);
- replacing omega-6 oils and butter with olive oil;
- eating omega-3 rich seafood; and
- taking supplemental omega-3 fats.

The glycemic index is a measurement of how quickly and to what extent a food raises blood sugar and insulin levels. Generally, the more processed the food, the higher its glycemic index; but this isn't always the case. For example, a fresh boiled potato has a glycemic index of 70 on the glucose standard chart, but spaghetti has a glycemic index of 50. White rice is a 72, white bread a 69, and pure fructose (fruit sugar) is only a 20! (I don't recommend foods high in fructose; research indicates that eating a lot of fructose causes elevations in bad cholesterol.)

In the appendices section you will find a list of common vegetables and fruits and their glycemic index values. Photocopy it and use it to make your shopping lists and plan your meals. Choose primarily foods with a glycemic index below 50—such as leafy greens like spinach or collards, or tomatoes, apples, or berries—and you will be well on your way to eating yourself young. Your blood glucose levels will remain right around 100. Your cholesterol and triglycerides will drop. So will your blood pressure.

Life is short, but it does offer a lot of delicious things to eat. Moderation and awareness are key. When you have a sandwich, don't eat—or save till later—the top slice of bread. When you eat cake, have a small slice instead of a huge chunk. If you partake of rice or crackers, just have a small serving. Split restaurant entreés with a companion.

Here's what you need to know to stay on a low-glycemic diet:

- At every meal, consume a lean protein source, in a serving about the size of your palm, with a generous serving of a low-GI vegetable or fruit. Add a small portion of a good fat; olive oil is best.
- Eating protein or fat along with a high-GI food will lower the glycemic index of the meal as a whole.
- If you're snacking, lower its glycemic index with a low-GI food.
- When you long for high-GI, carbohydrate-rich foods, remember that this is an evolutionary imperative you are fighting and that the human body is programmed at the genetic level to eat as much carbohydrate as possible to produce and store fat in case of a future famine. Acknowledge this, forgive yourself, and then say, "No thanks" to more carbohydrates.

When possible, avoid sandwiches, choosing instead a salad with a vinaigrette dressing, topped with lean chicken or fish. You can add whole grains such as rice, lentils, or beans. The awareness point here is, don't bring about an insulin surge. If you don't raise insulin, you won't glycate; you won't store fat but will instead metabolize it. And you won't be hungry.

Savor sweets when you have them. But if you're a person who can't resist overindulging, for whom one sweet turns into two and then three and then a sugar fest, you should avoid them completely. It's just not worth it.

OPTIMAL EATING GUIDELINES, PART TWO: LOW-CALORIE

Eating for optimal life span and quality of life involves systematically consuming 30-40 percent fewer calories than you would eat if you were to eat as much as you wanted to while still getting all the vitamins and minerals you need. This amounts to about 1,100 calories per day for women and 1,400 for men.

I recommend about 1,500 calories a day for women and 1,850-2,250 for men because restriction beyond this is just too hard to maintain and can have consequences. Aside from the fact that it is likely to make you completely miserable, extreme caloric restriction decreases production of growth and sex hormones and increases production of cortisol.

Every time you choose to eat sensibly and moderately, you are prevailing over a deeply ingrained instinct to eat as much as you can. Again, acknowledge this accomplishment and tell your instincts that food will always be available. Get a general idea of your intake of calories but don't be obsessive about it. Be conscious of your portions. Any movement toward eating less food on a daily basis will improve your chances of living past one hundred with all your faculties intact.

Keep in mind that beverages—even healthy ones—carry calories. A glass of juice or wine or a sweet coffee drink can contain 100 or more calories of quickly metabolized sugars.

Often we think we need food when we really need water. Cleanse yourself with an inner shower! Drink a lot of water, at least six eight- to twelve-ounce glasses a day.

You'll feel an increase in energy, your skin will be more supple, and you'll retain less water as your body won't feel the need to hang on to it with a steady supply coming in. Adequate water also helps to flush toxins and keeps the bowels moving smoothly. For every workout you do, drink an extra glass of water.

BROCCOLI, CAULIFLOWER, CABBAGE, TOMATOES: FOODS TO INCLUDE

Broccoli, cauliflower, cabbage, kale, and brussels sprouts—the cruciferous vegetables—are the richest natural sources of indole-3-carbinol (I3C), a nutrient that seems to help prevent cancers stimulated by estrogen. Broccoli sprouts are an especially rich source of I3C.

I3C's action in the body is similar to that of the breast cancer drug tamoxifen. Like the breast cancer drug tamoxifen, it converts estradiol (the most powerful cancer-promoting form of estrogen) to 2-OHE (a weaker form that does not promote cancer) and decreases levels of 16 alpha-hydroxyestrone, a metabolite of estrogen associated with breast and endometrial cancers.

Where women can benefit from foods rich in I3C, both men and women can benefit from foods rich in the carotenoid lycopene. Higher levels of lycopene in blood and tissues are associated with decreased risk of cancers of both the prostate gland and lungs. Lycopene inhibits human cancer cells in at least three ways—interfering with cellular signals that promote their growth, slowing their proliferation by up regulating the gene concerned, and finally, killing them (apoptosis).

The best way to add lycopene to your diet is by eating tomatoes cooked in olive oil. Try tossing tomato chunks in olive oil, sprinkle with herbs and a dash of salt, and roast in a 350-degree oven until very soft. Use them to top fish or chicken or try them with fresh mozzarella or whole grains.

GINGER AND CURCUMIN: ANTI-INFLAMMATORY HERBS

The closely related herbs ginger and curcumin are the most effective natural anti-inflammatory agents known. Ginger is pale yellow, pungent to the taste, and comes from the root of the ginger plant while curcumin is bright yellow-orange, has a milder flavor and is made from the root of the turmeric plant. The two oldest medical systems, Chinese and Ayurvedic (East Indian), have used both for millennia.

Ginger and curcumin are rich in potent antioxidants. They contain plant chemicals that alter eicosanoid production, reducing inflammation like the popular nonsteroidal, anti-inflammatory drugs. But unlike drugs, they don't target single biochemical reactions, so their effects are more balanced, and they don't have side effects. A growing body of research confirms that these herbs are excellent natural medicines for cancer prevention, chronic inflammation, and pain.

Both turmeric and ginger are used in curry, a blend of herbs and spices that is a mainstay of Asian cuisine. I encourage you to partake liberally of them, in your food or as supplements.

FOR WHAT WE ARE ABOUT TO RECEIVE, WE GIVE THANKS: CONSCIOUS EATING

The key to eating less than your instincts tell you to eat is to eat consciously. Engage your awareness and acknowledge your soul each and every time you eat—whether you are wolfing down a donut in your car on your way to work or sitting down to a beautiful meal with your family.

> ### Eggs from Happy Chickens, Milk from Happy Cows
>
> Thich Nhat Hanh is a Vietnamese Buddhist monk, author, poet, teacher, and Nobel Peace Prize nominee. In his book Anger: Wisdom for Cooling the Flames, he describes how the foods we choose to eat can powerfully affect our emotions and how our awareness suffers when we ignore these emotions. He writes that the way we grow food and the food we choose to eat make a difference, both in our own lives and in the world at large. By choosing to eat humanely raised animals and organically grown crops, we can reduce the suffering of those animals and lessen the negative environmental impacts of modern-day ranching and agricultural practices. Hanh tells us that we need to eat "happy eggs from happy chickens . . . [and] milk that does not come from angry cows."

Don't punish yourself for dietary transgressions; just be aware of what you are eating and why you are eating it. Take small bites of food and chew for longer than you normally would, experiencing it fully and tasting it with your entire tongue. People almost never adequately chew their food! Slow down. Take a full, deep breath between bites. Slow down.

Offer grace each time you eat. Thank your Higher Power for the nourishment you are about to receive. Open your awareness to wherever that food came from, whether from a factory, a fertile field, or an animal that gave its life to nourish you. Wish for better nourishment for those who don't have enough. And remember that on our planet, where we have enough food to feed every person, millions still go hungry.

In life, there are two spaces: the sacred and the profane. When you eat, connect with the sacred. That animal gave its life so that you could eat.

That plant put forth its life energy and perhaps had its life ended so that you could be nourished. Don't take this for granted.

Recognize that someday, you will be food for the plants and animals. Holding this awareness makes any food "soul food."

CHAPTER FIVE

Nutritional Supplements: What You Need To Know

TODAY, VITAMINS AND mineral supplements are a very big, unregulated business. Industry statistics estimate that some 98.9 million American adults take one or more nutritional supplements. The Third National Health and Nutrition Examination Survey (NHANES III) found that 42.6 percent of non-Hispanic white Americans take at least one nutritional supplement.

Consumers in the United States and all over the world are taking supplements not to abate symptoms but rather to promote optimal health and prevent problems from arising in the first place. The question is, do they? We don't know. The evidence for all but a handful is equivocal. Some may even be harmful. In this chapter, I recommend only those nutrients that are known to be both safe and beneficial—not because of word of mouth, but because of solid scientific investigation.

Age Optimization calls for you to carefully choose everything you put into your body and maintain right relationship with all these substances. Supplementation should be evidence-based—meaning, it should be based on the results of independent clinical research—and not necessarily daily.

A study by Harvard researchers, published in a 2001 issue of the Journal of the American Medical Association, stated that *vitamin deficiency syndromes such as scurvy and beriberi are uncommon in Western societies. However, suboptimal intake of some vitamins, above levels causing classic vitamin deficiency, is a risk factor for chronic diseases and common in the general population, especially the elderly. Suboptimal folic acid levels, along with suboptimal levels of vitamins B6 and B12, are risk factors for cardiovascular disease, neural tube defects, and colon and breast cancer; low levels of vitamin D contribute to osteopenia and fractures; and low levels of the antioxidant vitamins (vitamins A, E, and C) may increase risk for several chronic diseases. Most people do not consume an optimal amount of all vitamins by diet alone. Pending strong evidence of effectiveness from randomized trials, it appears prudent for all adults to take vitamin supplements.*

Overall, the thrust of modern research indicates that a multivitamin/mineral is good insurance against premature aging and disease.

WHY WE MAY NEED TO SUPPLEMENT

Fewer than 29 percent of Americans eat five daily servings of vegetables and fruits—the foods densest in vitamin and mineral nutrition—with perhaps some 20 percent of Americans eating no fresh fruits or vegetables at all.

Nutritional analysis of modern fruits, vegetables, and grains reveals that these foods contain lower concentrations of nutrients than they did in the early 1960s, mostly due to soils having been depleted by modern growing techniques. Meats, dairy, and poultry have also lost much of their nutritional value. Factory-farmed cows and chickens eat even worse diets than most people do, and they too are what they eat.

One can only marvel that the human body can survive—even, for a short while, thrive—when fed nothing but processed garbage. Somehow it manages to extract and use whatever nutrients it can from whatever we put into it. And then we have the gall to be surprised when we end up sick and old before our time! Thank and honor your body by feeding it only good foods and nutrients.

BUYER BEWARE!

Consumers of all products need to exercise caution and good judgment. And this is doubly true with foods, drugs, and supplements.

Vitamins, minerals, and herbs are not as benign as many believe. They may have undergone little to no testing and are not regulated and labeled in a consistent way. When you go to buy one of the thousands of nutritional products available on the Internet and that line the shelves of stores, you have no proof that what you're buying is going to improve your health or even that the product contains what the label says it does. In several instances, supplements were tested by a neutral third party and found to contain only a fraction of the ingredients they were advertised to contain. In a few cases, nutritional products have been found to contain lead, mercury, or traces of prescription drugs.

You can find detailed information on nutritional supplements at Consumer Lab (www.consumerlab.com), which does independent testing of supplements submitted by their manufacturers. If you subscribe to their Web site, you can get a better grasp of which companies are offering quality products.

AGE OPTIMIZATION SUPPLEMENT RECOMMENDATIONS

I make a point of keeping up with the research on vitamins, minerals, and other nutrients to support optimal health and prevent disease. I only recommend supplements to my patients if they are strongly backed by high-quality scientific research published in peer-reviewed medical journals.

> ### A Note on Dosages
>
> Nutritional science is constantly moving forward and changing as new studies reveal new information on the optimal doses and combinations of nutrients. Therefore, I have chosen to suggest specific dosages only when the science is completely supportive of such a conclusion. Where a recommendation is not made, keep in mind that most quality supplements contain standard dosage levels of various nutrients that are adequate for

> the Age Optimization program and give dosage recommendations on their packaging.
>
> As you become supplement literate, stay abreast by reading the latest nutrition news in magazines, in the health section of your newspaper, and in the Web. Read what I have to say about each nutrient, study the literature if you wish, talk to your doctor about them, then create a plan that will work for you.

Take initiative and a proactive approach. Try a number of things, observe closely, and see what works for you. In a nutshell, "Patient, heal thyself!"

In the final analysis, perhaps the commonest hazard with supplements is just wasting time and money placing your faith in a worthless product when you could have placed that time, money, and faith in something that worked.

These are the ten nutritional supplements that I recommend you use. Contrary to most advice to take supplements daily without fail, I recommend a more moderate approach, taking these supplements two or three times a week.

If this list is shorter than you expected, don't be too surprised. I'm not in the vitamin business.

- Alpha lipoic acid
- Vitamin B6
- Vitamin B12
- Vitamin E
- Folate (folic acid)
- Vitamin D3 (1000-2000 mg) plus calcium and magnesium
- Chromium picolinate (before you eat something sweet or starchy)
- Coenzyme Q10 (daily)
- Lycopene
- Selenium (for men, to help protect the prostate)
- Omega-3 fatty acids from fish oil

Many of these nutrients can be found packaged in a multivitamin/mineral complex. Vitamin salespeople will try to convince you that you need a cabinet full of high-dose supplements. This just isn't true. We have ready access to highly nutritious food, and what we really need is better food with fewer empty calories. We need to quit eating crap that doesn't nourish us, not to pile a bunch of vitamin supplements on top of the crap.

Moderation is advisable with supplements, just as it is with food. Maintaining balance is much more health promoting than taking megadoses of this, that, or some other trendy new thing. Say "no thanks" to aggressive sales pitches for supplements, become informed, and make your own good choices.

Antioxidants: Team Players

To evaluate the effects of a nutrient on health and longevity, researchers give that nutrient—and only that nutrient—to the subjects in the study. But this methodology is inherently flawed: Foods typically contain more than just one kind of antioxidant, with the various types of antioxidants working together as electron donors and recipients. As noted earlier, a spent antioxidant becomes a harmful free radical. And so, in this unnatural "scientific" context, excessive amounts of free radicals can be created. This explains why some studies show that high doses of antioxidants administered in this manner can have adverse effects.

Taking a large dose of C occasionally to stave off illness or combat infection is fine; but ideally you would take it in combination with vitamin E, alpha lipoic acid, selenium, and lycopene.

VITAMINS: YOUR CELLS' METABOLIC MACHINERY

A vitamin is an organic compound (meaning that it contains carbon) that is used in small amounts by the body's metabolic (energy-producing) machinery. Most vitamins play multiple roles in the body. Several function as antioxidants, donating electrons to neutralize free radicals. The antioxidant nutrients also donate electrons to one another, reactivating antioxidant molecules that have "quenched" free radicals. Vitamins play many important roles, including promoting blood clotting, enhancing immune function, and maintaining the health of organs, bones, and skin. Vitamins E, C, D (as a companion to calcium), B6, B12, and folate are the vitamins I recommend.

Vitamin E is a fat-soluble antioxidant. Its main function is to prevent lipid peroxidation, the process where free radicals attack polyunsaturated fatty acids in cell membranes and damage the membranes. Some immune cells—those that produce a burst of free radicals when they engulf pathogens—require a lot of vitamin E. Preliminary research indicates that vitamin E helps prevent and delay the onset of coronary artery disease. Like vitamin C, E travels in the bloodstream and helps prevent the oxidation of bad LDL cholesterol.

Vitamin E appears also to support resistance against colds and flu. Influenza and pneumonia together constitute the fifth leading cause of death in the United States. The older you are, the more likely you are to become seriously ill with the flu.

Flu vaccines help some people; but older people, having weaker immune systems, tend not to respond as well. New flu strains, for which we don't have vaccines, commonly emerge. Two studies at the University of North Carolina found that a normally benign strain could mutate into a highly dangerous one that attacked the heart muscles of mice suffering from depleted selenium and vitamin E. And young mice eating depleted-selenium food developed much worse cases of the flu than the mice on normal diets did. The selenium-deficient mice also revealed much greater and longer-lasting lung inflammation.

I recommend natural vitamin E, which is sold as d-alpha tocopherol, or mixed tocopherols and tocotrienols (which can include alpha tocotrienols or alpha, beta, gamma, or delta tocopherols). Synthetic vitamin E (dl-alpha tocopherol) is not as active in the body.

Some research has found a pro-oxidant effect of doses of vitamin E above 200 IU daily, as well as a slightly increased risk of cardiovascular problems with high doses of this nutrient. Limit intake to 200 IU per day; you can take 400 IU every other day, or 800 IU once a week.

Vitamin D is not really a vitamin. It can be made in the skin during exposure to sunlight. Adequate vitamin D levels have been found to protect against many types of cancer (especially colorectal and breast cancers), autoimmune diseases, psychosis, diabetes and respiratory infections. Vitamin D is important for the incorporation of calcium, magnesium and other minerals into bones. And in the modern world with modern diets, almost no one gets enough vitamin D.

Since most of us spend most of our time indoors, and since dietary sources don't come close to fulfilling the body's need for vitamin D, supplementation is very important. Sunscreen blocks skin's vitamin D production, as does having naturally dark skin. Even those who do go outside in the sunshine without sunscreen for the 15 or so minutes per day required to make vitamin D may not make enough if they live in northern latitudes. Obesity and advancing age also reduce vitamin D production.

Take 1,000-2,000 IU per day of vitamin D3, the form of vitamin D best utilized by the body. Eat something that contains oil or fat when taking your vitamin D supplement to enhance absorption.

Vitamin C is a water-soluble antioxidant that also appears to support better immune system function. Take it in combination with vitamin E and alpha-lipoic acid to achieve a full spectrum of antioxidant protection; try up to 500 mg a few times a week.

B vitamins are depleted in modern processed foods. Without adequate B vitamins, the human body cannot detoxify its tissues, its energy wanes, and the skin becomes flaky or rashy. We lose some ability to absorb B vitamins as we age, with B-vitamin depletion being linked to dementia, depression, and mood disorders, as well as other conditions that strike the elderly. Lack of B vitamins has been linked strongly to increased risk of heart disease, some cancers, and Alzheimer's dementia.

B12, folate, and B6 are needed to break down homocysteine, an amino acid made in the body from proteins in the diet. Homocysteine can accumulate in the body when B vitamin intake is inadequate. High homocysteine directly damages blood vessel walls and is implicated in Alzheimer's and heart disease. Research has also linked osteoporosis, kidney failure, psychiatric disorders, and premenstrual syndrome to hyperhomocysteinemia (high levels of homocysteine due to insufficient B12, B6, and folate). Some health care professionals estimate that up to a third of people diagnosed with major depression have a measurable deficiency of folic acid.

B vitamins are found in leafy greens, nuts, seeds, and whole grains; but the refining of seeds and grains removes much of their B vitamin content. Although small amounts of B vitamins are added back into flour, the overall intake of B vitamins has fallen considerably since processed foods became the norm. B vitamin levels are reduced by stress and by many prescription medications.

Most multivitamins contain adequate amounts of these B vitamins: thiamin (vitamin B1), riboflavin (vitamin B2), niacin (vitamin B3), pantothenic acid (vitamin B5), and pyridoxine (vitamin B6). Some even contain enough vitamin B12, but for reasons I'll give later, people over the age of fifty seem to need a little extra.

In one fourteen-year-long study of 800,000 female subjects, those who took a daily multivitamin (containing folate) or ate diets rich in folate had the lowest incidence of heart disease. In another study, 101 men diagnosed with heart disease took folate, B6, and B12 supplements for four years. Ultrasound pictures showed that the plaque in the men's carotid arteries (the vessels that carry oxygen-rich blood up to the brain) had decreased in size, with those who began with the highest homocysteine levels seeing the greatest improvement.

If your multivitamin does not supply at least 50 mg of B6, 800 mcg of folate, and at least 100 mcg of B12 daily, use an extra B-complex supplement to round out your program. If you choose to take a B12 supplement, try a sublingual version, which you place beneath your tongue, where it's absorbed directly into the circulation. You can take up to 1,000 mg a day or two each week. (Extra B12 is stored in your liver.)

MINERALS: THE BODY ELECTRIC

Most people know how important electricity is to our world, but not many know that our bodies also run on electricity. The heart beats because of electrical current. The nerves fire because of electrical current. Muscles contract and release due to electrical current.

Minerals are inorganic substances that help create and alter the electrical currents that flow across cell membranes. The eighteen minerals needed for life also serve as structural building blocks of vitamins and hormones, and they influence immune function and the excretion of wastes. Calcium, magnesium, chromium picolinate, and selenium (for men) are the minerals I recommend.

Calcium does a great deal more than build bone. It plays a vital role in nerve cell transmission, the contraction and relaxation of muscle cells (including the heart muscle) and the constriction and expansion of blood vessel walls.

Osteoporosis Prevention

Most people think of osteoporosis as a disease that only strikes in old age. But bone loss begins long before the telltale signs of this disease—curved upper spine, stooping posture, deep bone pain, and high susceptibility to fractures—ever appear.

Adolescence and early adulthood are the prime times for the building of strong bones. If you don't protect your bones while you're still young, the damage will have already have been done by the time you reach late middle age.

Four out of every ten white women in America can expect to suffer a hip, spine, or forearm fracture once they have passed the age of sixty-five. Five of every ten will sustain small, painful spine fractures that will cause them to shrink in height. This is not only due to inadequate intake of calcium but also the combination of chronic, subclinical deficiencies in calcium, magnesium, vitamin D, and a few other trace minerals, coupled with inactivity and overconsumption of dietary protein and phosphoric acid from soft drinks. These deficiencies usually begin in young adulthood, so building strong bones should start at this time, and this will do more to prevent osteoporosis than any amount of calcium pills consumed after menopause.

To avoid osteoporosis, you should take not only calcium but also other minerals and vitamin D, and get plenty of exercise. Bio-identical hormone replacement therapy will also help minimize bone loss as you age—with estrogen and progesterone being particularly recommended for women.

Studies have demonstrated that calcium supplementation does more than help maintain bone density. Calcium also curbs weight gain, aids weight loss, reduces the risk of colon cancer, helps control hypertension, and relieves symptoms of premenstrual syndrome (PMS). One study even found that pregnant women who weren't meeting optimal calcium intake recommendations had higher levels of lead in their blood, posing potential harm to the nervous system of the developing fetus. The pregnant women's bones were demineralizing higher levels of lead in supplying nutrients for the baby's skeleton. Calcium supplements decreased the rate of demineralization and led to a drop in the subjects' blood lead levels.

Many forms of calcium are available. Check the label to see which kind you're getting. Your best values appear to be calcium citrate, calcium gluconate, or calcium malate. In each case, the calcium is chelated and thus better absorbed by the body. You can use hydroxyapatite or calcium hydrogen, but don't use oyster shell calcium because of the risk of mercury contamination and because this form of calcium is not as well absorbed.

The dairy industry seems to exploit every possible piece of pro-calcium research. But keep in mind that broccoli, kale, turnip greens, bok choy, collard greens, sardines, blackstrap molasses, almonds, and tofu processed with calcium salts are all great sources of calcium and have a good balance of calcium and magnesium. Plain, live-culture yogurt is another good source of calcium. It appears that calcium supplements work best when taken daily for an extended period.

Adults over fifty and pregnant or nursing women should get 1,200-1,600 mg/day. If you're under fifty, take at least 1,000 mg of calcium per day. Teens should take 1,300 mg/day, kids aged four to eight need 800 mg/day, and children under four should be given 500 mg/day. Many supplements contain both calcium and magnesium in a 2:1 ratio. If your multivitamin does not contain at least 400 IU of vitamin D, choose a calcium/magnesium supplement that also contains vitamin D3 (cholecalciferol).

Magnesium is a mineral that is even more deficient in the standard American diet than calcium. It participates in more than three hundred enzymatic reactions in the body, including those that manufacture fatty acids and proteins. Even small increases in magnesium intake can have large effects on the heart's ability to pump efficiently and regularly, and on the general health of the body's blood vessels. Magnesium plays a major role in maintaining proper arterial pressure, which explains why supplementing this mineral helps control hypertension. Because magnesium regulates heart rhythm and relaxes constricted blood vessels, it is often infused intravenously during cardiac emergencies.

According to the Institute for Functional Medicine, magnesium can help to improve the following conditions: angina, asthma, cardiovascular disease, congestive heart failure, diabetes, fatigue, fibromyalgia, glaucoma, hypertension, insulin resistance, irregular heartbeat (cardiac arrhythmia), osteoporosis, and premenstrual syndrome. Because this mineral prevents the constriction of blood vessels in the brain, it is indicated for complications due to stroke and other cerebral accidents.

Take magnesium as magnesium citrate, magnesium glycinate, or magnesium malate, or as a mixture of these and other chelates. Don't take more than 600 mg of magnesium a day unless advised to do so by a physician.

Selenium is a trace mineral that works with vitamin E. The two together have much greater antioxidant capacity than either alone. Selenium appears particularly effective at preventing cancer, most notably cancer of the prostate, the most common cancer in men.

Accordingly, men with higher selenium levels show a decreased risk of prostate cancer. A study performed at the University of Arizona at Tucson compared two groups of men. The members of one group took 200 mcg of selenium a day while those in the other group took a daily placebo pill. The selenium group was diagnosed with 77 cancers during the follow-up period, while the placebo group had 119. Deaths from cancer varied similarly: The selenium group had twenty-nine deaths, with the placebo group, fifty-seven. The figures were statistically significant and the results very encouraging, so much so that the study was halted early to allow all subjects to start taking daily selenium.

Other research suggests that supplemental selenium has a protective effect against cancers of the breast, colon, and skin. Add 200 mcg of selenium to your supplement plan if it isn't already in your multivitamin.

OTHER NUTRIENTS: COENZYMES, CAROTENOIDS, AND FATTY ACIDS

In this category: alpha lipoic acid (ALA), acetyl-L-carnitine, coenzyme Q10 (coQ10), lycopene, and omega-3 fatty acids. ALA and CoQ10 are made in body cells, and can be supplemented to promote better health and longevity; omega-3 fats, as you already recognize if you have read this far, support less inflammation and better heart health. Lycopene is a carotenoid, like beta-carotene; it has been found to have powerful anti-cancer effects.

Coenzyme Q10 is made within each and every animal and human cell. Its scientific name is ubiquinone because of its ubiquitous nature. Its main role is to help power the cells' tiny energy-producing engines called mitochondria.

CoQ10 is an antioxidant that protects against lipid and protein peroxidation (the attacking of fats and proteins by free radicals) and donates electrons to regenerate spent vitamin E. This nutrient decreases the stickiness of blood, making dangerous clotting less likely, and increases the flow of blood to the heart muscles.

Our peak serum levels of coQ10 occur in our late teens or early twenties, and by the time we are putting on a party hat for our eightieth birthday bash, our coQ10 levels have most likely fallen by 65 percent or more. CoQ10 can be depleted also by poor eating, stress, strenuous exercise, and some prescription drugs—most notably, the statin drugs prescribed to millions to lower their cholesterol.

Coenzyme Q10 has been used in Japan since 1974 as a medical treatment for cardiovascular disease. An estimated 12 million Japanese take it on a regular basis. Many clinical studies of coQ10 have shown improvement in congestive heart failure patients. The support for its use as an adjuvant therapy (a treatment that accompanies the pharmaceutical drugs usually prescribed for a condition) is so strong and its safety profile so excellent that some experts feel it's a travesty that every heart disease patient is not on coQ10.

Although statins are marvelous drugs that lower cholesterol and reduce inflammation, some research suggests that they don't prolong life as we might expect. This is most likely due to the coQ10 depletion factor. Every person on statins should use this supplement!

Another study suggests that coQ10 can aid in fat loss. Many overweight people have slower metabolic rates, and coQ10 speeds metabolic rate at the cellular level. Obese subjects were given low-calorie diets plus 100 mg of coQ10 or a placebo for eight to nine weeks. Members of the coQ10 group lost an average of thirty pounds while placebo group members lost only thirteen.

Periodontal disease can be a major issue for older people, and coenzyme Q10 is an effective therapy for this too.

Use an encapsulated coQ10 supplement dissolved in oil (which enhances absorption). Or open up a capsule of dry coQ10 and sprinkle the powder on nut butter or butter.

Alpha lipoic acid (ALA) is an antioxidant nutrient made in the body. Adding extra in supplement form appears to be especially important for people who are insulin resistant or diabetic, but the research suggests that it may be useful for anyone wishing to slow the aging process at the cellular level.

Researchers from the University of California at Berkeley and the Children's Hospital of Oakland Research Institute found that a combination of two substances—alpha lipoic acid and acetyl-L-carnitine—had astonishing youth-restoring effects on aged rats. Bruce Ames, one of the scientists on the UC Berkeley team, put it this way: "With the two supplements together, these old rats got up and did the macarena." The carnitine enhanced mitochondrial function, increasing cellular energy, and the ALA appeared to mop up the extra free radicals created by this revving of the cellular engines.

Dr. Ames and his colleagues fed ALA and acetyl-L-carnitine to rats that were twenty to twenty-four months old (the equivalent of seventy-five to eighty human years), and they behaved like rats less than half their chronological ages. Old rats given the two supplements showed improvements in memory, mitochondrial function, and cellular antioxidant activity.

Age-related memory loss is believed to be at least partly due to free-radical damage to the brain. In one of the UC Berkeley studies, the researchers showed that alpha lipoic acid plus acetyl-L-carnitine decreased oxidative damage and structural decay in the hippocampus, the part of the brain most affected by Alzheimer's disease.

The importance of ALA in biological systems has been known since the 1950s. It's endogenous, meaning that it's made in the body, and like coQ10 is necessary for the proper transformation of food into energy at the cellular level. Alpha lipoic acid is one of the most potent antioxidants known, but it only "does its magic" when a certain minimal amount is available to the cells. When enough ALA is available, it deactivates free radicals and donates electrons to spent antioxidants and thus rejuvenates them.

Alpha lipoic acid regenerates vitamin E, vitamin C, and glutathione. Glutathione is another endogenous antioxidant essential for cellular detoxification, especially in the liver. People with cancer, autoimmune disease, AIDS, and other diseases have been found to have low levels of glutathione. ALA reliably raises glutathione levels in the cells and also inhibits glycation, the process by which sugars bind to cellular proteins. Glycated proteins produce free radicals at a rate fifty times that of non-glycated proteins.

The accumulation of heavy metals—including lead, mercury, aluminum, and iron—is almost certainly a significant cause of premature aging. These metals enhance the production of free radicals, and the body tends to lose its ability to efficiently excrete them as we grow older. ALA is a chelator of heavy metals, meaning that it binds to them and extracts them from the tissues. The metals become water soluble and can be flushed through the urinary tract.

Neuropathy (nerve damage) commonly accompanies diabetes. This condition is caused by free-radical damage to nerves and is characterized by symptoms like sharp pain, prickling, and numbness in the lower legs and feet. A collaboration between scientists at the Mayo Clinic and in Russia found that alpha lipoic acid supplementation "significantly and rapidly reduces the frequency and severity of symptoms of the most common kind of diabetic neuropathy." Alpha lipoic acid was found to directly improve nerve conduction. Today ALA is commonly used in Germany for the treatment of complications related to diabetes.

Sciatica, a source of serious back pain, especially in diabetics, is one such condition. A study performed at the University of Iowa found that the small blood vessels that fed the sciatic nerves of diabetic rats tend to clamp down, reducing oxygen availability. This, in turn, causes pain and nerve damage. In diabetic rats pretreated with ALA, the sciatic blood vessels opened up and allowed increased blood to flow to the nerves.

A Canadian research group gave daily ALA to a group of rats genetically predisposed to diabetes and hypertension. All experimental animals were fed a diet containing 10 percent pure glucose, with those not getting ALA showing a 29 percent increase in blood pressure, a 30 percent increase in blood glucose, a 22 percent increase in a particular type of free radical, a 286 percent increase in insulin, a 408 percent increase in insulin resistance, and a 63 percent rise in glycated protein. The rats given ALA showed much smaller increases in insulin levels and insulin resistance, and no increases in glycation and the types of free radicals measured in the study.

Using mice genetically altered to develop Alzheimer's disease, another research group studied the effects of ALA and another nutrient called N-acetyl-cysteine on memory impairment and oxidative brain stress. The two supplements enhanced the rodents' performance on a series of memory tests and decreased the oxidation of fats and proteins in their brains.

Yet another study, from the Linus Pauling Institute, found that topical application of alpha lipoic acid reduced the oxidation caused by exposure to ultraviolet radiation. Researchers reported that a combination of ALA and vitamin C increased the synthesis of nitric oxide in the human aorta, a major blood vessel. This is because nitric oxide relaxes blood vessel walls, counteracting the constriction and clogging that lead to heart attacks and strokes.

Anywhere from 100-600 mg per day of ALA can be used safely. You can use this amount daily or a few days a week.

Acetyl-L-Carnitine (ALC) was one of the two supplements that got aged rats to get up and boogie at UC Berkeley. Here's why:

During the process of cellular metabolism, acetyl groups—fragments of the carbohydrates and fats we burn for fuel—must pass across the membrane of the mitochondria to be transformed into energy. Acetyl-L-carnitine carries these acetyl groups to where they are needed.

This nutrient has also been found to possess remarkable neuroprotective properties, meaning it guards nerve cells against damage by oxidation and other kinds of stress. One study published in the journal *Clinical Cancer Research* found that ALC helped prevent the often-severe and permanent nerve damage caused by the chemotherapy drugs Paclitaxel and Cisplatin.

Several studies have found acetyl-L-carnitine protecting against injury to neurons (nervous-system cells) in both humans and animals. Others have shown that ALC can help prevent or slow the progression of Alzheimer's disease, conclusions supported by magnetic resonance imagery (MRI) studies of subjects before and after ALC administration.

Consider these additional research findings. ALC

- bolsters various aspects of immune system functioning;
- decreases the number of errors and improves many aspects of performance, including hand-eye coordination, reaction time, and learning speed in young women administered complex video game tests;
- elevates mood in both AAMI patients and healthy individuals;
- enhances the body's dopamine chemistry (dopamine being a feel-good brain chemical) by boosting its secretion, increasing its ability to bind to its receptor sites, and retarding the receptors' decline in Parkinson's sufferers;
- helps infertile couples wishing to have children by raising the man's sperm count, improving sperm shape, and improving sperm motility;
- improves creativity, memory, and attention span in those suffering from age-associated memory impairment (AAMI);
- increases the distance that people afflicted with intermittent claudication (a painful condition resulting from plaque buildup in the blood vessels of the legs) can walk without pain;
- maintains vision by protecting the neurons of the optic nerve;
- promotes alertness and hand-eye coordination;

- shortens reaction time in those with cerebral insufficiency (decreased blood flow to the brain).

In animal studies, ALC has been found to improve nerve conductivity, speed nerve conduction velocity (the speed at which nerve impulses travel), and thicken the protective myelin sheaths that cover the nerves in hyperglycemic mice; increase running speed; raise plasma testosterone levels; reduce stress-induced release of cortisol.

ALC is not cheap, but it's a remarkable supplement and well worth the cost. Use 500 mg two to four times daily.

OMEGA-3 FATTY ACID SUPPLEMENTS

Choose a supplement made from fish body oils that delivers 1,000 to 2,500 mg per day of the omega-3 fat, docosahexaenoic acid (DHA) from anchovy, salmon, or sardine oils. The average fish oil supplement will provide 120 mg DHA and 180 mg eicosapentaenoic acid (EPA) per gram of oil, which will entail taking at least ten 1-gram capsules each day. This isn't hard to achieve, if you take a few morning, noon, and night.

Higher-potency supplements will have higher concentrations of DHA and EPA per gram, so if you're not into swallowing a lot of pills, high-potency supplements are your best bet.

Your fish oil supplement should be molecularly distilled to remove toxins. It should also contain an antioxidant like vitamin E or rosemary oil to counter oxidation.

SOME CONCLUDING REMARKS ON NUTRITIONAL SUPPLEMENTATION

Human beings are not machines. We don't come off an assembly line, and each of us has different requirements for life's necessities, including nutrition, love, touch, and laughter, among others. No two people have the exact same vitamin and mineral requirements. Each person's need for supplements depends on his or her physiology, gender, age, genetic makeup, stress level, and day-to-day activities.

The guidelines I provide in this chapter are general, and each person will need to use discernment and "tweak" them for maximal benefit. Lab testing for vitamin levels in your body is available today, and using these test results will enable you to fine-tune the vitamins and amounts of vitamins you take.

CHAPTER SIX

Going Steady: Hormone Replacement for Men

Note to women: Don't skip ahead just yet as the first section of this chapter is for you too. I will let you know when you should turn to chapter 7, which is just for you.

ESTROGEN, PROGESTERONE, AND testosterone (if you are a woman) and testosterone (if you are a man) are the biochemicals that make you attractive to the opposite sex, that fuel your sex drive, and that orchestrate the symphony of reproduction. And they all dwindle as you age. Most experts agree that the drop in hormone production with aging is directly attributable to this reduction in sex hormone activity. The good news is that you can replace these hormones, bringing your body's levels back up to those it had in your fortieth year.

Although they are usually called sex hormones, these hormones also work in ways that have nothing to do with sexuality or procreation. They also affect the function of the circulatory system, bones, muscles, and brain. Nearly every cell in your body has receptor sites for at least one of these hormones.

In this chapter for men, we'll look at the hormone that makes men masculine: testosterone. The following chapter (chapter 7) is for women. Just as the female psyche and physiology are more complex than those of the male, so is the maintenance of female hormonal balance. It involves all three hormones—estrogen, progesterone, and testosterone—hormones whose levels fluctuate on a monthly basis and over the course of a woman's reproductive life.

When levels of these hormones drop, you can replace them. Usually, to do this safely and effectively, we use bio-identical hormones—hormone supplements containing hormones that exactly match the body's naturally produced hormones.

WHAT ARE HORMONES?

Hormones exert a profound influence over the workings of the body and in turn are influenced by the state of the body and its environment. They play major roles in our thoughts, feelings, and actions.

Hormones work on the cellular level. They attach to specific receptor sites on specific cells and, in so doing, trigger changes in the activities of those cells. You can think of hormones as the "on" switches that initiate various cellular processes. Groups of cells make up organs, groups of organs make up organ systems, and a group of organ systems makes up the body as a whole. Hormones transmit information and energy throughout the body, maintaining homeostasis: an ever-changing state of balance that enables the body to adapt to any and all changes in its internal and external environments.

Here's how they work:

1. The body senses something and notifies the brain.
2. The brain evaluates the message from the body and judges it important.
3. The brain informs the body of this important thing.
4. The brain responds by secreting hormones from a part of itself called the hypothalamus into the bloodstream.
5. These nervous system hormones activate the body's other endocrine glands, which in turn secrete more hormones as needed.

The adrenal glands, walnut-sized organs that sit atop the kidneys, produce testosterone and DHEA in both sexes. They also produce small amounts of estrogen and progesterone. Men's testicles make testosterone. Women's ovaries make the hormones estrogen and progesterone. Growth hormone is produced by the pituitary gland in the brain. All these glands lose steam as you pass through your fifth decade of life. Some fail gradually (such as the testicles, adrenals, and pituitary) while others crap out more suddenly (the ovaries, at menopause). Testosterone, estrogen, and progesterone can be safely replaced.

Hormone testing and replacement can seem expensive, but keep in mind that these tests and therapies are cheap compared to the cost of bypass surgery, hip replacement, dialysis, and other procedures used to rescue people who have not been proactive about protecting their health. In past, insurance covered every penny of these surgeries and therapies, but nowadays patients must bear an increasing portion of the expense themselves.

The only real solution to the health care crisis is Age Optimization. Eating well and exercising are great ways to start, but hormone replacement will make a major difference for a lot of people by enhancing their quality of life and extending their life spans.

HORMONE TESTING

When I provide hormone replacement for a patient, I take a moderate approach and attempt to restore hormone levels to about the 65th percentile for a thirty-nine-year-old. I don't ever try to produce a higher-than-average level of hormones, as too much can be more dangerous than too little.

I advise hormone replacement patients to get tested every two or three months to make sure the dosages are right. And even if they are right today, they will need to be modified to accommodate changes the patients will experience as they move through the years. This is particularly true for men taking testosterone. I like to test for total and free testosterone every three to four months and then in the mornings only, as the tests will not produce accurate results if given at any other time.

Women readers, if you aren't interested in reading about hormone replacement for men, you can move on to the next chapter.

MALE MENOPAUSE: MYTH OR REALITY?

Do men have a "menopause"? Technically, no, but we are finding that men in fact do experience a similar transition, though a more subtle one, where their testosterone, DHEA, and growth hormone production falls and their estrogen, insulin, and cortisol rises. A better word for the male change of life is andropause, although the term has yet to catch on.

Menopause is a more dramatic transition characterized by more pronounced symptoms, reflecting the complete cessation of progesterone and estrogen production. Because this change is relatively abrupt, its effects are more obvious. The more gradual and less dramatic andropause has only recently been acknowledged as something that can be controlled with hormone replacement therapy.

Hormone replacement is exactly that—hormone replacement. It's only recommended for those who have overt, easily identifiable symptoms of deficiency, or whose deficiency has been confirmed through laboratory testing. If your tests reveal healthy levels of hormones, you should not supplement.

TESTOSTERONE BASICS

The link between testosterone and male vigor was first noted in ancient Greece. Pure testosterone became available in 1935. In 1940 and 1944, the *Journal of the American Medical Association* published articles on the use of testosterone for the treatment of the "male climacteric."

Research has continued to demonstrate that testosterone is an effective treatment for angina (heart pains caused by clogged blood vessels) and claudication, and that it can decrease body fat and enhance muscle and bone mass in aging men. Further studies have shown that testosterone replacement can lower cholesterol, normalize abnormal heart rhythms, and help reverse the onset of type 2 diabetes.

Testosterone is made in the adrenal glands of both sexes and in the testicles of the male. It begins to decrease around age fifty and continues to do so at the rate of about 1.5 percent per year. It increases libido, boosts production of growth hormone, builds muscle and bone mass, reduces fat mass, regulates insulin sensitivity, lowers blood sugar, lowers "bad" LDL cholesterol, boosts energy, and enhances mood.

Symptoms of low testosterone include anxiety, depression, fat increase, impotence (in men), insomnia, irritability, loss of body hair on chest and genitals and unwanted growth of body hair elsewhere, loss of libido, low energy, and muscle loss.

Diabetic men see an early decline in testosterone production, and more than 50 percent of them have low testosterone levels. When a man comes to me with erectile dysfunction (ED) and tells me that he's tried Viagra or Cialis to no avail, he is almost always overweight and diabetic. These men need to lose some weight and gain some testosterone, and when they do, the impotence drugs will usually work.

Testosterone, estrogen, and progesterone are all steroid hormones; but don't confuse them with the synthetic, patentable anabolic steroids taken by bodybuilders and athletes. The term "steroid" simply means the hormone is made from cholesterol. DHEA and cortisol, for example, are also steroid hormones. Anabolic steroids have received much bad publicity in recent years, and by now most people know that they are dangerous.

FREE VS. BOUND

Testosterone bound to another molecule cannot be used by the body as it attaches to receptor sites only in its free form. In this case, the decline in free testosterone is more pronounced than the overall decrease in testosterone production.

One molecule that testosterone binds to is sex hormone binding globulin (SHBG), also known as just globulin. If you go to a physician for what you imagine to be symptoms of dwindling testosterone and he tells you that your total testosterone levels are just fine, this is why: You are making enough testosterone, but too much of it is bound to SHBG and is unavailable. Testosterone not bound to SHBG is free testosterone, and this is what does all of testosterone's jobs in your body.

Approximately 30 percent of men in their sixties and 80 percent of men over eighty are believed to have a low free-testosterone index. You will need to ask your doctor to test both your total and free testosterone levels to get an accurate picture of your overall testosterone activity.

BENEFITS TO HEART AND BONE HEALTH

Men with low testosterone are more likely to have high blood pressure, high triglyceride levels, and low HDL, all of which are well-established risk factors for cardiovascular disease. Replacement of this hormone in deficient men decreases waist-to-hip ratio (also a good indicator of cardiovascular risk) and restores more healthy levels of total cholesterol and LDL cholesterol.

The heart muscle contains many testosterone receptors; a weakened heart muscle in an aging man often suggests testosterone deficiency. Testosterone maintains protein synthesis in muscle throughout the body and promotes the dilation (opening) of the arteries that feed this muscle with oxygenated blood. In one study, testosterone supplementation improved blood flow to the heart muscle by 68.8 percent!

TESTOSTERONE AND THE BRAIN

Alzheimer's disease is on the rise as the population ages, but little is known about its cause. Similarly, no effective treatment has been discovered to slow or halt the progression of the disease. More minor loss of memory and thinking power is an annoyance faced by most aging men. Testosterone could prove to be a man's best shot at preventing Alzheimer's. This hormone decreases the formation of beta-amyloid, a protein that accumulates in the brains of people with Alzheimer's disease.

Both testosterone and estradiol (a form of estrogen) have *neuroexcitatory* effects, meaning that they enhance the firing of neurons in the brain. This is why replacing these hormones helps to reverse the age-related phenomenon of absentmindedness, lessening the incidence of "senior moments."

TESTOSTERONE AND YOUR PROSTATE

Most published studies show that serum testosterone levels *don't* affect the risk of prostate cancer. In twenty-one of twenty-seven published studies, no increase in prostate cancer risk was found with testosterone supplementation. One study was inconclusive, with the other five finding small increases in risk. Further studies have reported that men receiving testosterone supplementation had a slightly increased risk of prostate gland enlargement, known formally as *benign prostatic hypertrophy* (BPH).

Although most men who develop prostate cancer have *low* levels of free testosterone, a certain amount of caution is indicated because if a man has undetected prostate cancer, testosterone can cause it to undergo a growth spurt. I always do prostate-specific antigen (PSA) testing before I give a man testosterone, and I repeat the test every thirty to forty-five days while he is taking it. If his PSA levels rise suddenly, I know that his prostate needs attention.

Most prostate cancer cell lines require testosterone to proliferate. The increased aromatization of testosterone to estrogen may be one mitigating factor (see the coming section on aromatization for more on this); when estrogen binds to globulin in the prostate gland, prostate cells proliferate. In BPH, free testosterone levels show a downward trend while estrogen stays the same or increases.

Men with BPH can ask their urologists about taking Proscar or Avodart, both alpha-reductase inhibitors that counteract the formation of dihydrotestosterone (DHT) in the prostate. All evidence indicates that this is the form of testosterone that causes BPH.

Some men see their DHT levels rise steeply when they start to use testosterone. This is another reason to monitor hormone levels with blood testing. If you happen to be one of these men, you might need to take an alpha-reductase inhibitor along with your testosterone. DHT has also been linked to male pattern baldness, but again, Proscar can be used. It's commonly applied directly to the scalp as the drug called Propecia.

Herbs for Prostate Enlargement

A substantial amount of research has shown that benign prostate enlargement can be controlled with the herbs saw palmetto, pygeum, and nettle. These herbal supplements can relieve BPH symptoms like urinary urgency, inability to completely void the bladder, and increased frequency of urination. The most obvious symptom is a sudden need to get up several times a night to urinate.

Try one, two, or all three herbs at once. Of the three, saw palmetto has the best documented therapeutic effects.

- Nettle: 300-600 mg twice daily
- Pygeum: 100 mg once daily or 50 mg twice daily
- Saw palmetto (85-95 percent fats/sterols): 160 mg twice daily
- Zinc/copper chelate: 80-90 mg of zinc daily
- A zinc/copper chelate containing 80-90 mg of zinc taken daily will also help maintain good prostate health.

AROMATIZATION ISSUES (WHICH HAVE NOTHING TO DO WITH COLOGNE)

In a small subset of men, supplemental testosterone is transformed—*aromatized*—into estradiol, a form of the female hormone estrogen. Aromatase enzymes make this conversion in the fat cells in both sexes—this is how fat cells make estrogen—and excessive aromatization can, in some men, turn testosterone into estrogen. When these men are given testosterone, they may start to grow breasts. Increased estrogen levels also increase the risk of prostate cancer.

Fortunately, with frequent hormone testing, we can take appropriate action. A drug named Arimidex (generic name, anastrozole) is used to treat women with breast cancer. It turns off aromatization enzymes and shuts down estrogen production in fat cells. It will also stop aromatization in men who are taking testosterone. Its most common side effects in women are weakness or sleepiness, but these occur only very rarely in men. Arimidex is expensive—a couple hundred dollars a month—but if you're a man whose testosterone is changing into estrogen and you wish to use testosterone, Arimidex is your only option.

DO YOU NEED SUPPLEMENTAL TESTOSTERONE?

If you are fifty or older and have more than two or three of the symptoms of low testosterone noted in this chapter (anxiety, depression, fat increase, impotence [in men], insomnia, irritability, loss of body hair on chest and genitals and unwanted growth of body hair elsewhere, loss of libido, low energy, and muscle loss), have your level of testosterone measured. If your test comes back below 700, seriously consider a trial of testosterone replacement therapy.

My male patients who use testosterone experience huge improvements in their energy level and physique. Libido, potency, reaction time, and endurance usually improve, as do blood sugar and insulin levels. Some men will get oily skin or acne, with a few (only about 10 percent) experiencing shrinkage of the testicles—a side effect that is reversed by lowering the dose or stopping testosterone therapy.

Taking *too much* testosterone can cause libido to spiral out of control. It can also increase heart attack risk and cause irritability, aggression, oily skin and acne, and water retention.

Bio-identical testosterone is available. Many doctors will prescribe it in the form of gels, patches, lozenges, subcutaneous pellets (rice-grain-sized pellets inserted just beneath the skin, which dissolve slowly over the course of weeks or months), or creams.

I usually prescribe injectable, oil-based testosterone cypionate. This is not a bio-identical form of testosterone, but you cannot inject bio-identical testosterone or take it orally, as it can't be properly used by the body unless absorbed through skin or mucous membranes. I've found it close enough to do the job without untoward effects. It is injected intramuscularly with a fine-gauge needle, which allows the hormone to diffuse slowly into the circulation and maintain a consistent level. Testosterone can also be taken orally, in pill form, but I do not recommend this form. It tends to raise testosterone levels too high and then drop them too low, and it can damage the liver.

Talk with your doctor, who you will need to prescribe the hormone, about which form will be best for you. *You cannot take testosterone without a physician's prescription.* No over-the-counter product can legally contain testosterone, bio-identical or otherwise.

CHAPTER SEVEN

You Make Me Feel Like An Optimal Woman: Estrogens, Progesterone, And Testosterone

MANY WONDERFUL WOMEN I have known enter a marvelous time of spiritual exploration in their menopausal years: deepening relationships, doing good work, savoring life's pleasures, and letting the "small stuff" slide away to make room for what is truly important to them.

Unfortunately, for many women, this time of life may also include hot flashes, night sweats, diminished libido and reduced pleasure during sex, mental fogginess, irritability, insomnia, and decrease in vaginal tone and lubrication. It usually marks the beginning of accelerated skin aging and a jump in the risk of cancer and heart disease.

These are all issues that can be at least partially remedied with the judicious use of hormone replacement therapy, along with plenty of exercise and a low-glycemic diet that prevents glycation and keeps insulin levels steady.

For decades, medicine believed that replacing estrogen with a concoction of estrogens derived from the urine of pregnant mares and a synthetic form of the hormone progesterone (called a *progestin*) would relieve menopausal symptoms and prevent heart disease, age-related cognitive problems, colon cancer, and osteoporosis, while causing no increase in breast cancer risk. Since the turn of the new millennium, we have known better.

BREAST CANCER RISK AND HORMONE REPLACEMENT THERAPY

In 1997, a study was published in *JAMA* (the *Journal of the American Medical Association*) that raised concerns about a possible HRT-breast cancer connection. The researchers evaluated data from fifty-one previous studies and found a trend toward increased risk of breast cancer in women who underwent standard estrogen/progestin replacement therapy—usually, with a combination horse estrogen/progestin pill called Prempro or another combination of horse estrogens (Premarin) and a progestin—after menopause.

Until late 2002, despite much evidence that traditional hormone replacement therapy did more harm than good, widespread use of Premarin by menopausal women continued. Then the Women's Health Initiative (WHI) study results were published, causing even staunch supporters of traditional HRT drugs to do a double take. Millions of women stopped taking the drug, all at the same time. And for many of them, menopause symptoms like hot flashes, vaginal dryness, mental fog, mood swings, and insomnia rushed back with a vengeance.

The WHI was the largest randomized prospective study in the history of conventional hormone replacement. It involved 16,608 healthy menopausal women from forty different locations in the United States. The study was halted three years early because researchers found that HRT posed serious health risks to the subjects.

Roughly half the women took Prempro; the other half, a placebo (dummy) pill. During the 5.2 years of the study, an increase in breast cancers was found, with eight additional cases per 10,000 Prempro-taking women. The Prempro group experienced significantly more heart attacks and blood clots. Any benefits of the drug (small decrease in risk of colon cancer and fractures due to osteoporosis) were outweighed by its liabilities. Women who had no risk of uterine cancer because they'd had hysterectomies took only Premarin (no progestin), and they were the only HRT-using group that did not show higher rates of heart attack and blood clots than the group on placebo.

The women involved in the WHI were at least sixty by the time they began their hormone replacement program. By that time, it was probably too little and too late. Their bodies had been hormone-deprived for a decade by then. Women who were taking statin drugs or baby aspirin on a regular basis were about half as likely to have deep-vein thrombosis (blood clots) than women who weren't, but this wasn't factored into the statistical analysis of the data in this study.

Despite its flaws, the WHI study was the push that sent the traditional HRT boulder past the pinnacle and down the hill. It is now common knowledge that Premarin plus progestins should *not* be used routinely or long-term to prevent age-related diseases. Temporary use of these drugs to combat some menopause symptoms—hot flashes, vaginal dryness, and night sweats—is advised for some women. *Bio-identical* estrogens, progesterone, and testosterone, which so far appear to be safer and just as effective, are a much better alternative for women whose hormone levels are low and uncomfortable symptoms are a problem.

THE BIO-IDENTICAL DIFFERENCE

The results of the WHI were no great surprise to anyone who had been following the research on hormone replacement therapy. Slight increases in breast cancer, blood clots, and heart disease make perfect sense when you consider how synthetic progestins and Premarin work in the body. So do mood changes and irritability often linked to use of traditional HRT.

What the medical establishment has until now mostly refused to acknowledge is that safe alternatives to these drugs are available. These alternatives have been studied for some time now—at least as long as the more commercially popular progestins and Premarin combinations. These alternatives are natural, bio-identical versions of the hormones made in a woman's body, the same hormones that decrease at menopause.

When you put non-bio-identical hormones into the human body—either synthetic progestins or hormones from pregnant horse urine—they don't work the same as our natural versions do. These pharmaceutical hormones can "gum up" our cellular machinery. They have *estrogenic* and *progesterone-like* effects on cells, but their activity is far from identical to that of the body's own natural hormones.

Bio-identical hormones are derived from plants like Mexican wild yam or soy. They are made in facilities certified by the USP (United States Pharmacopoeia), just like any drug you might take. Molecules from these plants are molecularly "tweaked" until they are identical to the hormones found in the human body.

Premarin is a concoction of several varieties of estrogen, derived from the urine of pregnant mares. It could be loosely termed *natural* but is certainly not bio-identical. Progestins are brand-new substances made from molecules having actions *similar* to those of natural progesterone; they are not progesterone although most scientific research papers use these terms interchangeably.

With regard to the female hormones estrogen and progesterone, bio-identical versions are turning out to be safer and just as effective. Why does medicine continue to develop and use synthetics? Because natural products and bio-identical products cannot be patented, and patented products command much higher profit margins.

Another wrinkle is that a natural or bio-identical equivalent can be patented if it is delivered to the body in a new way. For example, bio-identical progesterone, when taken orally, has to be *micronized*—reduced to particles only a few microns in size—and this process makes it patentable. Additionally, natural or bio-identical products can be *combined* in a novel, patentable way. A case in point is Premarin, which contains all natural (if partially equine) estrogens.

Without the exclusive rights that patents bring, drug company profit margins would tumble. Many popular Western drugs sell at profit margins over 99 percent! So the drug companies push only what they can patent and ensure that only synthetics undergo large-scale, properly funded studies and get FDA approval. Drug companies' publicity machines only push their products, and so it's little surprise that most people don't know they have other options. Now that synthetic HRT has fallen out of favor, bio-identical progesterone and estrogens could finally get the attention and respect they deserve.

Bio-identical hormones exactly match the hormone molecules made in the human body. Your body cannot tell these hormones from the real deal. For women, bio-identical hormone replacement after menopause may include estradiol, progesterone, and testosterone.

COULD YOU BENEFIT FROM BIO-IDENTICAL HRT?

Ideally, you should begin having your baseline hormone levels measured long before you hit menopause. Then check them once a year or so and start to replace hormones (with safe bio-identical equivalents) as soon as you see a downward slide in your numbers. If you wait until your fifties, you could lose a lot of ground that you could have held had you begun your program sooner.

On the other hand, if you are already into your fifties or beyond, there is probably no reason to avoid bio-identical estradiol, progesterone, or testosterone, unless you have had estrogen-receptor positive breast cancer, ovarian cancer, or endometrial cancer. (If you have had any of these diagnoses, consider bio-identical HRT very carefully, with the help of your physician. Women who have had breast cancer or any other type of reproductive system cancer that rules out their use of estrogen replacement can use progesterone alone and derive much benefit from it.

Estrogen comes in three "flavors"—*estradiol, estrone,* and *estriol.* These versions of estrogen differ in their potencies and biochemical actions in the body. Estradiol is the most commonly prescribed bio-identical estrogen, and it is administered via patch, subcutaneous (under the skin) pellet, cream, or sublingual lozenge or drops. You cannot take bio-identical estrogens orally; they will be completely broken down by the liver before they can reach your tissues.

Research has shown that women who start Prempro late in life may actually have adverse effects to the heart, but these effects are due to inflammation caused by oral estrogens' effect on the liver. Using estrogens that are not swallowed but delivered by creams, patches, lozenges, drops, or tiny pellets inserted just beneath the skin will circumvent this effect on the liver, allowing any woman who's low on estrogen to use it without risk to her heart.

TOO MUCH ESTROGEN...

The risks of low progesterone are most evident when coupled with normal or above-normal levels of estrogen. This is often the case with women who experience an uncomfortable transition into menopause. As ovulation happens less often during the premenopausal years, progesterone levels drop but estrogen keeps cranking.

During the years just before menopause, estrogen often ends up *high* relative to progesterone as ovulation slows down and stops altogether. A low progesterone-to-estrogen ratio in the years before menopause can lead to many different problems, including infertility, polycystic ovary syndrome (which causes infertility, weight gain, acne, and facial hair growth), repeated miscarriages, thyroid problems, and uterine fibroids (benign tumors that can grow very large and cause many of the six hundred thousand hysterectomies performed each year in the United States). Also linked to a low progesterone-to-estrogen ratio: decreased sex drive, fibrocystic breast disease, increased risk of breast and uterine cancer, heart disease, and osteoporosis.

In some premenopausal women, progesterone production is normal but estrogen is high, due to use of birth control pills or to obesity or overweight (fat cells make estrogen).

This imbalance between progesterone and estrogen is now widely known as *estrogen dominance*, a term created by John Lee, M.D. If you want a more in-depth explanation of estrogen dominance and the problems it can cause, I highly recommend the books Dr. Lee wrote with journalist Virginia Hopkins: *What Your Doctor May Not Tell You About Menopause*, *What Your Doctor May Not Tell You About Premenopause*, and *What Your Doctor May Not Tell You About Breast Cancer*.

Too much progesterone relative to estrogen, which is a very unlikely situation in anyone who isn't slathering herself with progesterone cream, can cause sleepiness or low energy.

Progesterone replacement, when needed, aids in building bone, burning more fat for energy, enhancing libido, and improving mood. By far, the most popular route for progesterone replacement is transdermal cream, which is available over the counter. Because there's no guarantee that a product not prescribed by a doctor will contain the hormone it says it contains on the label, I recommend you go to your physician and have him or her send your prescription to a compounding pharmacy.

Progesterone can't be administered through a pellet or patch because the dose required is too high. This hormone can be prescribed orally as micronized progesterone, also known as Prometrium. The patients I see are usually very happy with it. It can relieve bloating and other estrogen dominance-related complaints almost immediately and aids sound sleep when taken in the hour before bed.

... OR NOT ENOUGH ESTROGEN?

Despite what doctors consider to be optimal ranges for hormones, each person's hormonal balance is unique. If, for example, levels of one hormone are high, a seemingly "normal" level of another hormone can be low. The range of so-called normal hormone levels are enormous. This is why, although hormone level testing is important, looking for *symptoms* that suggest a need for hormone balancing is equally crucial for an optimized state of physical and psychological well-being during the years around, during, and following menopause.

Symptoms like vaginal atrophy, hot flashes, urinary incontinence, uterine prolapse (where the uterus literally begins to turn inside out due to lack of tone), vaginal dryness, and night sweats in menopausal women nearly always have an easily identifiable cause: low levels of estrogen. Long-term low estrogen also has been found to increase risk of Alzheimer's, heart disease, and osteoporosis.

IF YOU USE ESTROGEN, YOU *MUST* USE PROGESTERONE

Estrogen should never be used without progesterone, even by women who have had hysterectomies, as these two hormones balance the effects of one another in the body. Blood vessel health, nervous system health, and bone health all improve when both hormones are supplemented judiciously.

You can, however, use progesterone without estrogen. Estrogen production doesn't completely cease at menopause because it is also made in fat cells through the action of aromatase. Additionally, progesterone "awakens" estrogen receptor sites, enhancing the action of existing estrogen.

TESTOSTERONE: GET YOUR MOTOR RUNNING

Is sex important to you? If it is, you have something in common with the majority of participants in a study called the National Social Life, Health and Aging Project (NSHAP) found that sexuality is an important issue for many people in their fifties, sixties, seventies, and eighties. This study of about three thousand American adults found a close connection between sexual activity and health, with more and better sexual activity reflective of better health.

Now the cause-and-effect equation could go either way here—better overall health could improve sexual health, or better sexual health could improve overall health. Either way, you have to admit that sex, when it's good and when you want it, is a quick ticket to deep, soulful awareness. It can be a meditation on life, death, birth, and relationship that enhances our sensual enjoyment of each day. Sexual energy is not something to be given up on lightly. It is a powerful source of intimacy and life force.

In the NSHAP survey, which was published in the *Journal of the American Medical Association* in 2007, nearly half of those who remained sexually active reported at least one sexual problem that posed an obstacle to satisfying sexual intimacy. This is a major reason why we have testosterone, estrogen, and progesterone replacement for women; testosterone for men; and Viagra and other erectile dysfunction drugs (more on these medications in chapter 9).

Some women find that estrogen replacement therapy further decreases their libido instead of reviving it. Estrogen replacement can cause a rise in sex hormone binding globulin (SHBG), a protein that renders sex hormones circulating in the bloodstream inactive. More SHBG decreases free testosterone in particular, diminishing libido and health in general. Adding a little testosterone to the mix can take care of the problem.

Testosterone is produced in a woman's body during her fertile years. Women produce only a fraction of what men do, with premenopausal women making only about 3/10 of a milligram a day. (Men can make as much as seven milligrams daily.) Still, a small amount of testosterone goes a long way.

Just days before ovulation, along with her estrogen levels, a woman's testosterone levels surge, and this probably explains why a woman's sexual desire increases at this time of the month. Giving estrogen and testosterone together appears to be the best way to restore lost libido in postmenopausal women.

Women have testosterone receptors in their nipples, clitoris, vagina, . . . and brains. If testosterone production falls, those receptors are starved for stimulation; it follows that adding testosterone back into the picture will get your motor running again!

Testosterone will not cause women to grow facial or body hair, and it won't cause clitoral enlargement or deepening of your voice—unless you take too much. When I recommend testosterone for women, it's usually in the form of a cream containing 1-3 percent testosterone, applied in very small amounts to the clitoris three times a week at bedtime.

A testosterone patch for women should hit the market sometime soon; I have also heard good things about subcutaneous pellets of testosterone, which are only the size of a grain of rice and are inserted in the physician's office through a one-fourth-inch incision that can be closed with a small Band-Aid.

Short-term Benefits of Bio-Identical HRT for Women

The effects of this type of hormone replacement will vary, but most women can expect to experience at least some of the following:

- Better sleep
- Improved insulin sensitivity
- Improved mood

- Improved psychological well-being and energy
- Improved thyroid function
- Improvement in fat-to-lean mass
- Improvement in motor stability
- Improvement in vision
- Increased ability to think
- Increased alertness
- Increased sex drive
- Increased sexual responsiveness (in one study, women on testosterone and estrogen showed an 80 percent improvement in libido!)
- Lowered blood sugar
- Relief from hot flashes and other menopausal symptoms
- Thickening and increased sensitivity of the nipples
- Thickening and strengthening of the skin (including the vaginal walls)

LONG-TERM BENEFITS OF BIO-IDENTICAL HRT FOR WOMEN

Many long-term benefits of bio-identical supplementation have been identified in research on the subject. The later you start, the more these conditions may progress by the time you begin with bio-identical HRT; but it appears that women can still benefit even if they start late in life.

Estradiol is known to protect against Alzheimer's disease. Replacing this hormone also helps women who complain of "brain fog" during and after menopause because it has a stimulating effect on the central nervous system. Estrogens also protect against cancer of the colon.

Along with progesterone, estradiol preserves bone mass and lessens the likelihood of hip fractures. Estrogen and progesterone work cooperatively to build and maintain bone in the female skeleton. An eighty-year-old woman not on hormones or other bone-building drugs may have lost about 50 percent of her bone mass. Twenty-five percent of women aged sixty to eighty incur a hip or vertebral fracture. As elsewhere, individual health and exercise habits make a big difference, but all evidence indicates that a regimen of estrogen plus progesterone beginning around menopause can significantly decrease this bone loss. Testosterone also appears to play a role in promoting production of new bone in women.

Replacing deficient estrogen is associated with improvements in several risk factors for heart attack. Estrogen replacement therapy has been found to improve the integrity of the *endothelium*, the inner lining of the blood vessels. It increases the diameter of blood vessels, which improves blood flow and enhances the pliability of the valves in the heart. The largest studies on the subject found a 35-50 percent reduction in coronary artery disease risk with estrogen replacement—that's estrogen only, without *progestins*.

From the available evidence—including a lack of increased heart attack risk in the estrogen-only arm of the WHI study—it's reasonable to conclude that the increases in heart disease risk in women on conventional HRT are due to the effects of progestins. Available evidence suggests that bio-identical progesterone is good for the heart, but the progestins constrict blood vessels, contributing to heart attack and blood clotting.

ESTROGEN AND BREAST CANCER

Many women shy away from estrogen replacement because of links between Premarin and breast cancer. I cannot say I blame them, as the evidence linking the two seems strong at first glance. However, *bio-identical* estrogen, given to an estrogen-deficient woman in doses that approximate levels seen in a healthy thirty-nine-year-old, has not been found to cause cancer. Most studies show that estrogen replacement *protects* women against colon and ovarian cancers. Using natural progesterone along with the estrogen will counteract the growth-promoting quality of estrogen.

If you are a woman over the age of forty, get your screening mammograms without fail, whether you use bio-identical HRT or not. Begin regular colon cancer screenings and continue with your Pap tests on schedule. Early detection really does save lives.

Along with the use of estrogens and progesterone together, I recommend that my female patients take indole-3-carbinol to prevent breast cancer. (It also helps to prevent prostate cancer in men.) This compound is found most abundantly in broccoli but is also available as a supplement. I-3-C affects the metabolism of estrogen to reduce the undesirable growth-promoting effects of this class of hormones in the body.

Should You Avoid Estrogen Replacement Altogether?

If you have any of the following symptoms, use progesterone only, under the guidance of a physician:

- Current or past breast cancer
- Current or past circulatory disease involving blood clots
- Damage from diabetes to the kidney, nervous system, or vision
- History of jaundice related to oral contraceptives
- Hypertension (over 160/100)
- Liver disease
- Migraines related to the menstrual cycle
- Smoking habit
- Structural abnormalities in the heart (making clots more likely)

If you are obese or overweight, you probably only need progesterone, unless you have severe menopausal symptoms.

Avoid taking estrogen if you plan to have major surgery requiring extended bed rest. Major surgery increases the chances of clot formation, and patients are advised to stop taking estrogen four weeks prior to surgery.

HOW TO OBTAIN AND USE SUPPLEMENTAL HORMONES

Women can have their estrogen, progesterone, and testosterone levels measured as soon as they start to experience menopausal symptoms or—if they don't suffer any discomfort during the change—once they are sure their periods have stopped. Hormone levels can be tested well before menopause by women who are experiencing extreme menstrual symptoms, irritability, infertility, or other "perimenopausal" symptoms as described in Chapter Seven. The best resources I know of for salivary hormone tests—the most accurate test for measuring estrogens, testosterone, and progesterone—are the following:

- *http://www.virginiahopkinstestkits.com/*, the Web site and store of Virginia Hopkins, who coauthored Dr. John Lee's books; and
- *http://www.zrtlab.com/*, the Web site of biochemist and saliva testing expert David Zava, Ph.D.

Although you do not need a physician's requisition to take a salivary hormone test, you will need the guidance of a physician to make the best possible use of natural hormones. While bio-identical versions are safer than synthetics, most of them are only available by prescription.

Progesterone is the exception (aside from Prometrium, the micronized progesterone pill). If you choose to use progesterone cream to supplement this hormone, I recommend that you ask your doctor for a prescription version to be made by a compounding pharmacist, or ask for an over-the-counter brand you can trust. Do not use any OTC cream that contains a mishmosh of herbs (none of these have been shown to go into the skin and be transformed into any hormone) or that claims to contain estrogens or "estrogenic herbs." Bio-identical estrogen is sold only by prescription. Any vendor of a cream that bills itself as a source of bio-identical estrogen that you can purchase without a prescription isn't giving you the straight story about its product.

While using natural hormones, take note of any side effects, which could indicate that your dose is too high or too low. Have your levels checked regularly to be sure they stay within the appropriate ranges. You could be challenged to find a doctor who will prescribe natural hormones, but the number of physicians willing to do so is on the rise.

Insurance might not cover these treatments, but be aware that HRT will probably save you much money during the remainder of your life—not to mention worry, anguish, pain, and heartache—in helping to prevent the ailments that can ruin your final years. And the improvements you will see in your energy level, your libido, and your overall health will further sweeten the deal.

When to begin bio-identical HRT? In my practice, I recommend that women

- *begin using progesterone monthly, starting on the fifteenth day of the menstrual cycle and stopping just before menstruation, starting in their late thirties or early forties if hormone tests show low levels.* Women can continue this pattern through and following menopause. I usually prescribe oral micronized progesterone, but creams can also be used successfully—just make sure to have a follow-up test so that you know it's getting your hormone levels to the best place for you. Apply enough each day to give your body 15-30 mg of the hormone, using it for only three weeks of each month. For dosages and counsel for the various "female problems," such as uterine fibroids, breast fibrocysts, infertility, and breast cancer, read the *What Your Doctor May Not Tell You* books. Much has been written about natural progesterone, but theirs were the first books on the subject and are the most thorough and easy to understand.
- *Begin to use estradiol as soon as tests show that their natural production of estrogens falls, or as soon as menopausal symptoms begin to show up.* I usually prescribe transdermal estradiol in a cream form, but patches and pellets work well for many women. I don't always give testosterone or estrogen, but I never give estrogen without progesterone.
- *If test results demonstrate low testosterone, add a natural testosterone cream (from a compounding pharmacist), which soaks into the skin and slowly introduces the hormone into the circulation.* Dosages will vary greatly from person to person, depending on hormone levels at the outset of supplementation, and can change over time. The bio-identical cream might not be enough for you if your testosterone is really low. When your test results come back, talk with your doctor about which form will be best for your needs.

There are many individual variations on these themes. Depending on a woman's symptoms and her hormone-level test results, I might recommend only oral progesterone and estradiol cream applied directly to the vaginal mucosa; or only transdermal testosterone for application directly to the clitoris, a tiny dab once daily, three to seven days a week. The latter approach hasn't been studied on a large scale, but my patients give me favorable reports, saying that it greatly enhances their sexual responsiveness—an effect of testosterone awakening the nerve endings. This is a safe practice as long as the dose is kept small.

I advise you to repeat the hormone-level tests every two to three months to make sure the doses are right. Yours will need to be adjusted to reflect the body changes that come as you move through the years. See appendix 2, Lab Testing, for standard hormone levels.

CHAPTER EIGHT

A Delicate Balance: Cortisol, DHEA, Melatonin, Thyroid Hormone, and HGH

WHETHER YOU ARE male or female, the hormones covered in this chapter are not as critical as the sex hormones. But because they interact with the sex hormones and because they affect your moods, emotions, the aging of your body, and your overall health and quality of life, you should still know a bit about them. You may or may not choose to investigate whether replacing any of these hormones is a good idea in your personal plan, or you may simply leave this chapter with an understanding of how to optimize your body's own natural balance of these hormones.

Our hormones are complex chemicals that exert dramatic effects on how our body feels to us, our mood, and our day-to-day experiences. They are powerful agents that act quickly—unlike nutritional supplements, which can take days, weeks, or months to make a perceptible difference in our health and well-being.

This chapter will keep things simple. I'll give you information about what each hormone is, what it does, its risks and benefits, and how to judge whether you may wish to consider using it to optimize your age.

DEHYDROEPIANDROSTERONE (DHEA)

As a supplemental hormone, DHEA has fallen in and out of favor over the years. It enters individual cells and is transformed into estrogen, testosterone, or one of several other steroid hormones, a process influenced by a number of factors.

Dehydroepiandrosterone is an adrenal steroid, like testosterone and estrogen. It is the most abundant adrenal steroid, and is produced in the adrenal glands and testicles. Like many hormones, DHEA is produced in small quantities in childhood and begins to rise at puberty, with the highest levels occurring during the early twenties. Each year after your twenty-fifth birthday, DHEA blood levels drop by about 2 percent. Still, the levels can vary greatly over the course of an individual's lifetime and, similarly, from person to person.

Studies have found that for some people whose DHEA levels are low, supplemental DHEA renews energy and vigor remarkably; others have suggested risks such as increased estrogen levels in some users. Disease and chronic stress impact DHEA levels. The hundreds of studies that have examined the relationships between disease and DHEA production have found that when illness strikes, DHEA levels are low. They are especially low in people with AIDS, diabetes, Alzheimer's disease, the autoimmune disease lupus, chronic fatigue syndrome, heart disease, and cancer. High alcohol consumption, obesity, smoking, certain medications, and problems with thyroid function can also lower DHEA levels.

DHEA is often called the "mother hormone" because it is the precursor from which most of the other steroid hormones are made. It is actually weakly androgenic (masculinizing). Men make more DHEA than women.

What are the benefits of DHEA?

Feelings of well-being are strongly correlated with high DHEA concentrations. Studies on rodents have demonstrated that DHEA is *neuroexcitatory*, like estradiol and testosterone: it stimulates brain functioning and also appears to protect the nervous system against age-related deterioration. Studies on

DHEA's ability to prevent Alzheimer's disease and other forms of senile dementia have been promising.

Libido is significantly affected by DHEA levels, particularly in women. Current research is also examining DHEA replacement as a treatment for erectile dysfunction (ED), and results here have been promising as well. Most clinical subjects, both male and female, report that it greatly improves their mood and rekindles their sex drive. It's also a good antioxidant.

DHEA replacement has been found to improve immune function in both immunocompromised people (particularly those with AIDS) and in people with autoimmune disease (especially lupus). Studies have found that the antibody response of older people to flu vaccination is even improved with supplemental DHEA.

DHEA is a precursor for testosterone, estrogen, androstenedione, cortisol, progesterone, and aldosterone; but it's also important in its own right. In lab animals, DHEA appears to have anti-cancer properties. It inhibits the activity of an enzyme, *glucose-6-phosphate dehydrogenase*, which in turn inhibits both the activation of carcinogens and the proliferation of cancer cells. It also slows the activity of an enzyme responsible for the production of the free radical that oxidizes LDL cholesterol in the bloodstream. This bad cholesterol, when oxidized, is more likely to form lesions (atherosclerotic plaque) in the arteries that can lead to heart attack and stroke.

What are the risks of DHEA?

Women who use too much DHEA are at risk of masculinizing side effects, including acne, development of facial hair, and loss of scalp hair. These side effects can be quickly reversed, with no permanent harm done, by lowering the dose or ceasing DHEA therapy altogether.

If a man tends to aromatize testosterone into estrogen, chances are good that he'll do the same with DHEA. Some women's testosterone levels rise when they use DHEA; others see a rise in estrogens. When you use this hormone, it's difficult to know how it will be transformed in your body.

Who should consider trying DHEA replacement?

Around five thousand scientific studies have investigated this hormone, but its actions are still not well understood. We do know, however, that DHEA replacement can help men and women who are deficient.

A salivary hormone test will tell you whether your DHEA levels are low. Trying the hormone is a low-risk proposition since it is available over the counter. Start with a very low dose, especially if you are female, and work up to the dose recommended on the container for your age and gender. Repeat hormone tests (which will show you whether you are aromatizing DHEA to excess estrogens) or symptoms (such as scalp hair loss or facial hair growth in women) will show you whether this hormone is a good idea for you. You are unlikely to need DHEA before you are forty-five or older.

DHEA can provide a source of testosterone for women who need a little extra. They can derive considerable benefit from as little as 5 mg per day, but the usual dose is 25 mg per day. Some women are advised to take 25 mg every other day, often before bed.

CORTISOL: THE STRESS HORMONE

What is cortisol?

Cortisol is known as the "stress hormone." It is made in the body from DHEA. The amount of DHEA your body turns into cortisol strongly affects mood. Higher DHEA to cortisol brings about feelings of warmheartedness and contentment; a lower ratio seems to produce feelings of being "stressed-out." When individuals master biofeedback and other methods of transforming negative thoughts into positive ones, the DHEA-to-cortisol ratio rises.

Cortisol manages the body's long-term adaptation to stress. When we are faced with a stressful condition—including cold, hunger, injury, low blood pressure, surgery, infection, pain, inflammation, intense exercise, or just emotional stress—the adrenals are stimulated to release cortisol. This hormone increases blood sugar levels, raises blood pressure and heart rate, sends lots of blood to the muscles, slows blood flow to the digestive organs, and sharpens perception and reaction time. When cortisol rises to a certain level, the body's feedback system instructs the adrenals to stop producing it until the next stressful moment comes around.

The main job of cortisol is to increase the amount of sugars (glucose) circulating in the blood so that the brain and heart are continually fed. Glucose is the brain's preferred fuel, and cortisol is one tool the body uses to ensure that the brain always has enough of it. Cortisol must be present for growth hormone and glucagon to do their jobs of breaking down stored fat and carbohydrates.

Levels of cortisol can vary greatly between individuals. Production of cortisol is highest in the early morning (up to 23 mcg/dl in the bloodstream on average) and lowest around midnight (6 or fewer mcg/dl). People who have difficulty coping with stress have higher cortisol than people who adapt effectively to stressful circumstances.

What are the benefits/risks of cortisol?

The benefits of cortisol are also its risks. This hormone performs indispensable duties in the body, but in people who are under chronic stress and levels stay high, it can cause cardiovascular disease, weight gain in the midsection, and high blood sugars.

Cortisol is a key biochemical in the well-known fight-or-flight reaction to stress. The fight-or-flight response evolved to protect us when we're in a life-threatening situation. But people today are exposed to ongoing daily stresses that are not life-threatening and cannot be dealt with by either fighting or fleeing. Instead, we must use our brains instead of our bodies and handle the stress in a rational and constructive manner. Fight-or-flight served our ancestors well for millennia—through the first 98 percent of human history!—but today this response is obsolete and almost always inappropriate.

Under moderately stressful conditions—let's say, the average American adult's daily life—cortisol is continually secreted, which usually means that it's oversecreted. Eventually, the brain overrides the feedback mechanism designed to keep the cortisol level under control, and so it remains too high for too long. Add to this the fact that cortisol levels creep higher and higher as we age, and you can see how high cortisol contributes greatly to age-related health problems.

Stressed Out—and Don't Know It?

Stress in Western culture is often worn like a badge of honor. In my medical practice, I've found many a patient who is suffering from intense stress to the point of illness but still doesn't realize that stress is the problem. Sometimes the person just isn't ready to acknowledge this, choosing instead to focus on some other source.

Here are some signs that you might be more stressed than you realize:

- Absentmindedness
- Anxiety, irritability, and jumpiness
- Catching every illness that goes around
- Diarrhea
- Distractibility
- Erectile dysfunction
- Exhaustion
- Feeling that you're "missing out" because you aren't more "on top of things"
- Imagining terrifying things happening to you or your loved ones
- Infertility
- Menstrual problems
- Muscle tension (especially headaches and neck, shoulder, and back pains)
- Nagging self-doubt
- Shortness of breath
- Sweaty palms
- Unexplained nausea or upset stomach
- Unexplained skin problems

Coping effectively with stress is paramount for a long and healthy life. See the sidebar in chapter two entitled "Quick Checklist of Stress-coping Techniques," discussions of exercise, and the remainder of this chapter for advice on getting the stress monkey off your back.

One of cortisol's primary roles in the fight-or-flight response is to raise blood pressure. This improves the zebra's ability to escape a lion, but it doesn't help you when you're stuck in traffic or trying to meet a deadline at work.

Robert Sapolsky, a world-renowned neuroendocrinologist who teaches at Stanford University, studies the impact of stress on primates. He has found that chronic stress raises blood pressure and adversely affects the lining of the arteries and promotes atherosclerosis—the clogging of the arteries by cholesterol-filled plaque. Fatigue, emotional stress, and low social status have all been linked to increased risk of atherosclerosis due to high cortisol secretion.

Chronically high cortisol also eats away at the bones. One of the best known side effects of mainstream corticosteroid drugs (powerful synthetic versions of cortisol) is osteoporosis. High levels of natural cortisol can, over the years, have similar effects on bone density.

High cortisol also "turns down" the immune system, causing it to produce fewer of some types of immune cells. (The zebra running from the lion doesn't want to devote any energy to fighting off germs.) This increases the body's overall susceptibility to infectious diseases. Even inhaled steroids such as those used for asthma have this side effect, and yeast infections of the mouth and throat are common in asthma patients who use them. Cortisol overload also reduces growth hormone levels.

An extreme overload of cortisol, usually due to tumors in the adrenals or pituitary gland, causes Cushing's disease. Its signs are unmistakable: fat deposits collect on the torso while muscles in the arms and legs shrink, the buttocks and thighs grow thinner as the belly expands (does this sound like most of the men you see lined up at the all-you-can-eat buffet?), skin and bone both become thinner and more fragile, and blood pressure and blood sugar rise. In people who have much milder, but still chronic, elevations in cortisol levels, the effects are less extreme.

Even mildly high cortisol increases insulin, which increases appetite—for carbs especially—and packs pounds on your frame. For the zebra that just outran the lion, this mechanism is clearly adaptive as it replenishes the calories burned from fleeing the predator. For the harried working mother who just had a close call on the freeway, though, or who has had to take her toddler to the emergency room for stitches, it is not. Either way, the mother's appetite is going to increase.

High cortisol causes the body to store excess fuel as fat by raising insulin levels. Adding insult to injury is the fact that eating sugar makes cortisol rise. This means that those extra calories taken in during a cookie or ice cream binge will be stored in the body as fat.

Those suffering from dementia in general have higher ratios of cortisol to DHEA. Depression, anxiety, panic disorder, and alcoholism are further problems associated with excess cortisol. When cortisol is high, sex hormone levels fall. The last thing a zebra wants to do when being chased by a lion is procreate.

In chronic fatigue syndrome (CFS) and fibromyalgia, both DHEA and cortisol levels are low. Some theorize that these diseases result from *adrenal overload*—chronically overstressed adrenal glands that can no longer keep up with the demands of a stressful existence. Their production of steroids falls. A small, prescribed supplement might be necessary to help relieve symptoms of fibromyalgia or chronic fatigue.

How to keep cortisol levels in a healthy balance?

Controlling your daily cortisol levels isn't complicated, but it isn't easy, either. Knowing the damage that uncontrolled stress can do will help you to make stress relief a high priority. The relationship work I described in chapter two will help you to stay serene through the storms of life, and so will reframing stressful tasks as opportunities for meditation, chances to play, or challenges that will aid your growth.

A low-glycemic diet will prevent the insulin peaks and valleys that adversely affect cortisol levels. Some other things you can do to alleviate stress:

- Do something repetitive or artistic like draw, paint, scrapbook, or knit.
- Do something to enhance the beauty or peacefulness of your home.
- Take a yoga class or learn to practice yoga on your own.

- Try t'ai chi or chi gong—both ancient forms of meditative movement.
- Listen to soothing music or nature sounds.
- Perform volunteer work.
- Read a book.
- Spend quality time with someone you care about.
- Spend quiet time relaxing, meditating, or just being present and paying attention to your breath.
- Spend time outdoors in a place of natural beauty.
- Turn off the TV, computer, and radio.
- Garden or do yard work.
- Get some vigorous exercise.

Intense exercise burns off excess cortisol. If you are in generally good health, try a hard workout instead of three glasses of wine the next time you feel wound up from a hard day.

THYROID HORMONES

Thyroid hormone controls metabolism—the rate at which the body produces energy from food. It burns fat, reduces cholesterol, and supports the building of new protein molecules from amino acids, which in turn are used to build healthy new tissues. Low thyroid function causes metabolic rate to drop, and this is why hypothyroidism causes weight gain, cold hands and feet, fatigue, and depression. Goiter is seen in both hypo- and hyperthyroidism (where an overactive thyroid raises thyroid hormone levels too high). If a patient of mine shows signs of significant thyroid imbalance, I usually send him or her to an endocrinologist for therapy.

Thyroid replacement should never be used unless absolutely necessary. Once you start taking thyroid hormone, your body ceases to make it, and so you will never be able to stop taking it.

What are the risks of abnormal thyroid function?

Medications used to treat hypothyroidism—usually synthetic versions of thyroid hormone—are some of the top-selling prescription drugs on the market today. Low thyroid function is on the rise in aging people, and not every case of low thyroid function shows up in blood tests. This means that some people who could benefit from treatment of hypothyroidism don't get the right diagnosis. In women, hypothyroidism symptoms are often mistaken for those of menopause or premenstrual syndrome and can worsen the symptoms of both menopause and PMS.

As is the case with so many chronic diseases that afflict modern-day Westerners, thyroid diseases are only partially understood. The most widely accepted theory of thyroid imbalance says that it's an autoimmune response where the thyroid gland is attacked by the immune system. Some people have a genetic predisposition to thyroid disease. Autoimmune hypothyroidism is called *Hashimoto's thyroiditis*, and autoimmune hyperthyroidism is called *Graves' disease*.

Approximately 10 million Americans have low thyroid hormone levels. Only about 2 percent are men. Most are postmenopausal women. Overactive thyroid is a much rarer problem, usually caused by autoimmune disease or a thyroid tumor. Anyone with extreme jitters, dry skin, goiter (swelling of the thyroid gland), bulging eyes, rapid heartbeat, and unexplained weight loss should be evaluated for an overactive thyroid.

Many thyroid patients report disturbing changes in their bodies, emotions, interpersonal relationships, and ability to cope, even in instances of only mild thyroid imbalance. The symptoms of thyroid imbalance—the secreting of too little thyroid hormone (hypothyroidism) or too much (hyperthyroidism)—can cause depression and anxiety, which throw the thyroid gland even *further* out of whack, leading to even *more* depression and anxiety.

What are the signs of thyroid imbalance, and how is it treated?

Because most physicians are not trained to spot subtle signs of thyroid disease, mild thyroid dysfunction can be misdiagnosed as depression, anxiety, PMS, menopausal symptoms, or high cholesterol. *Exogenous* estrogens (those taken as supplements, as opposed to *endogenous* estrogens, which are made in the body) can have an aggravating effect on autoimmune thyroid disease, and drugs for anxiety or depression can worsen symptoms of thyroid imbalance.

In estrogen-dominant women, balancing estrogen with bio-identical progesterone is sometimes all that is required to clear up hypothyroid symptoms. Try this before trying thyroid hormone replacement.

> ### *Thyroid Hormone Testing*
>
> The standard blood test for thyroid imbalance is the TSH (thyroid-stimulating hormone) test. If thyroid hormones are low, TSH will read high as the hypothalamus sends more and more TSH into the circulation to try to jump-start the thyroid gland. If thyroid hormone level is high, the hypothalamus will reduce TSH production and the test results will reflect this change.
>
> Normal range for TSH is 0.4-5.0 milli-international units per liter. This range is so broad that a score at the bottom or top of "normal" could reflect thyroid activity that needs correction. In some cases, symptoms of thyroid imbalance persist despite normal blood test results. In these cases, the individuals might have a genetic factor that makes their thyroid hormones work less efficiently. Such people tend to respond well to thyroid hormone supplementation, which needs to be prescribed by a physician.

Synthetic thyroid hormone (levothyroxine, sold as Synthroid, Levothroid, and Levoxyl) is used to treat hypothyroidism. Unlike other synthetic hormones, synthetic thyroid hormone doesn't appear to have adverse effects.

HUMAN GROWTH HORMONE (HGH)

Adults with marked growth hormone deficiency—a rare condition—have slow metabolisms, thin skins, deteriorated muscles, more fat, kidney dysfunction, high cholesterol, high insulin, imbalanced moods, poor sleep, and shorter life spans. Severe growth hormone deficiency doubles the risk of death from cardiovascular disease. Accordingly, giving HGH-deficient patients supplemental HGH diminishes the risk, improving the pumping capacity of the heart and widening the diameter of blood vessels.

A lot of these changes are identical to the changes that occur with aging. And the average sixty-year-old person is *functionally deficient* in growth hormone. The pituitary gland, where HGH is made, makes about 14 percent less HGH each decade after production peaks during the full blush of young adulthood. This deficiency is not likely to cause overt or dangerous symptoms but does play a role in causing the body to age.

Growth hormone is *anabolic*, which means that it builds new healthy tissues to replace old, used-up tissues. It stimulates the creation of new bone, muscle, and connective tissue, supports the immune system, and causes the body to burn fat instead of storing it.

Human growth hormone (HGH) is an FDA-approved treatment for dwarfism and other kinds of small stature in children. Given by injection, this pituitary hormone can bring deficient children to full stature without side effects.

Adults who wish to slow the progression of aging are having impressive results with HGH. Those who use HGH replacement therapy report that they feel happier, more energetic, and less irritable and anxious. They also report feeling sharper—they think better, their attention spans increase, and their memory improves. Their skin appears more youthful, and keeping weight off becomes easier.

Who might benefit from HGH replacement?

Growth hormone replacement costs around $6,000 per year and has to be prescribed and monitored by a physician. It is injected once daily, in the morning, with a very fine-gauge needle (your doctor will show you how). Only very small amounts of the hormone are used. The goal, again, is to reproduce the levels found in a healthy thirty-nine-year-old. Proper dosage of supplemental HGH is essential. Giving too much growth hormone can actually raise insulin levels and promote insulin resistance, possibly leading to diabetes.

At this time, no bio-identical human growth hormone is available. The form currently used for replacement therapy is costly to make, and this is why it's so expensive. No product on any health food store shelf can contain growth hormone in any form that can actually get into your tissues and affect your cells. If you can't afford the real thing, you are better off allocating your resources toward other optimizing practices, not in purchasing some health-food-store junk that says it will raise your growth hormone levels.

You can enhance your body's natural production of HGH by

- *eating protein-rich foods*: Meals rich in protein cause human growth hormone levels to rise. Research indicates that supplemental amino acids, particularly arginine, can increase growth hormone production.
- *losing weight*: As overweight people make significantly less growth hormone than lean people, losing weight will cause HGH production to rise. When blood sugar drops, growth hormone surges. Remember that chronic underfeeding in animals raises their growth hormone levels, and they live longer and healthier lives. Periodic fasting will also boost HGH.
- *strength training*: Exercise that builds muscle stimulates higher growth hormone production.
- *taking melatonin*: In promoting sleep, melatonin enhances the production of HGH, whose production is highest at this time. More on this below.
- *using the right hormone replacement therapy*: Growth hormone production rises when testosterone and DHEA are replaced. Estradiol appears to reverse aging effects on HGH receptors and stimulates production of growth hormone-releasing hormone (GHRH) in the hypothalamus—the body's signal to the pituitary to release HGH.

MELATONIN: KEY AGE-OPTIMIZING HORMONE

Melatonin researchers Vladimir Lesnikov and William Regelson switched the pineal glands of ten young (three- to four-month-old) mice with those of ten aged (eighteen-month-old) mice, so that the young mice had old pineal glands and the old mice had young pineal glands. The old mice ended up living a little over thirty-five months while the young mice lived just under sixteen months!

The study's paper has a photograph of one of the young mice and one of the old mice together one year after their operations. They look exactly the same—same coat, skin, posture, and weight—despite their great age difference. (Every six months of a mouse's life is equivalent to twenty human years, so in human years the old mouse was more than four decades older.)

The pineal gland is a pea-sized gland in the brain that produces the hormone melatonin. This tiny gland is one of the most important organs in the human endocrine system. It serves as a biological clock, telling the body when it's night and when it's day, and triggering the production of specific hormones accordingly.

Melatonin is also thought to be triggered by specialized photoreceptors in the eyes. This hormone is also made by the walls of the gastrointestinal tract and in the retinas of the eyes. It makes you sleepy when night falls, regulates the function of the immune, digestive, and reproductive systems and the thyroid gland.

Melatonin production decreases naturally with passing years; by age sixty, we produce only half of what we did at twenty. Declining melatonin is closely associated with accelerated aging. This hormone is available over the counter as a supplement in most health food stores.

What are the benefits/risks of melatonin replacement?

Most of the studies of this versatile hormone have considered its potential as a natural, non-addictive sleep aid. The National Institutes of Health have invested millions of dollars in sleep research involving melatonin. In one study of melatonin and sleeping published in the October 2001 issue of the *Journal of Clinical Endocrinology and Metabolism,* researchers found that only 0.3 mg of melatonin taken a half hour before bedtime restored sound sleep in people over age fifty who had trouble getting a good night's rest.

Supplemental melatonin has been used to treat anxiety and depression. Evidence suggests that it may help those with Parkinson's disease and Alzheimer's disease. Melatonin might extend life span; low doses have lengthened the lives of lab animals by as much as 30 percent. And it's not just effective but very safe: test animals do not die from very high doses, and humans have taken up to 6,000 mg at a time with no side effects aside from sleepiness the following day.

High doses of melatonin have shown promise as a treatment for cancer and AIDS. Some human studies have demonstrated that high-dose melatonin (5-10 mg a day) benefits late-stage cancer patients. If you are undergoing cancer treatments and wish to try melatonin, discuss this with your oncologist.

In research by Russell J. Reiter, animals were given a dose of the poison safrole. Safrole does serious damage to the DNA of liver cells, often leading to cancer. Subjects given a small dose of melatonin along with the safrole had only 41 percent of the damage seen in the group that did not get the melatonin. With a larger dose, only 1 percent of the damage was found. Other research by Dr. Reiter found that when melatonin was administered to a group of animals exposed to what is normally a lethal dose of radiation, only half the number of animals died compared to the non-melatonin group.

Dozens of animal studies showing melatonin's anti-carcinogenic effects have been published. Melatonin clearly helps slow cancer growth in vitro (outside the body, when added to cancer cells in a petri dish) and in mice. Melatonin is a powerful antioxidant. It could also play a role in the intestines' absorption of zinc, a mineral particularly important for prostate health. Research has shown that supplemental melatonin normalizes zinc levels in people who are low on this mineral. Improved zinc levels could help explain melatonin's positive effects on immune function.

Low melatonin levels have been found in some forms of chronic depression, bipolar disorder (manic-depression), and chronic schizophrenia. In a study of people with seasonal depression—which is caused by too little exposure to sunlight—melatonin at night, along with bright light during the day, improved symptoms.

Melatonin tends to be low in migraine headache sufferers. Administering it during migraine attacks can both relieve the pain and decrease the number of migraines suffered. Studies by Italian researchers showed that melatonin supplements can improve immunity in both stressed-out individuals and the very old. Israeli and Swiss scientists gave melatonin to lab mice with encephalitis (a swelling of the brain caused by bacteria or viruses) and found the mice on melatonin were more than twice as likely to survive the often-fatal disease.

Who should try melatonin, and when?

Used occasionally, melatonin is a safe and highly effective natural sleeping pill—far superior to the addictive benzodiazepine drugs, which suppress melatonin production and decrease restorative REM sleep. Start with the lowest possible dose—a milligram or less—and work your way up until you find the dose that brings you sound sleep. Take a sublingual tablet (a fast-acting pill that dissolves beneath your tongue) a half hour before going to bed. If you find that your usual dose stops working after a while, don't take it for a week or so and start again rather than increasing the dose.

Use melatonin to offset jet lag or when you are having a tough time getting to sleep. If you have any condition listed in the previous section and want to explore using melatonin to help you back to health, refer to the book *Melatonin* by Russell J. Reiter and Jo Robinson, or to melatonin researcher Walter Pierpaoli's *The Melatonin Miracle*.

HORMONE REPLACEMENT IS NOT FOR EVERYBODY

Improvements in our understanding of how hormones optimize health and how they can be safely replaced when the body isn't producing enough of them let us move into our sixties, seventies, eighties, nineties, and beyond! in the best possible shape. Perhaps you are one of the lucky people who needs only a good food plan, some exercise, and a positive attitude to sail through the second half of your life looking and feeling great. You don't have to use hormones to achieve this, but for most of us, they help far more than they hurt.

CHAPTER NINE

The Age Optimization Workout

WHENEVER WE WORK our muscles and cardiovascular systems, we send the message to these parts of the body that their services are still needed. We're going to grab our lives by the horns, so to speak, and we need some muscles to do that!

Between the ages of twenty and forty, we lose 40 percent of our muscle mass as a natural consequence of aging. Fortunately, we do not lose the ability to *build* muscle. As long as testosterone levels are adequate, we aren't glycating proteins, and we eat a reasonable, nutrient-dense diet, we can still add a lot of muscle. Muscle gives us strength, dexterity, fluidity of movement, and resistance to injury and disease.

If you are already exercising regularly, this chapter will inform you about how exercise fits into the Age Optimization mind-set and how you might modify your present workout program for better results. If you are not exercising regularly, you might be hoping that I will share some secrets with you to transform you from the product of your current sporadic, dispirited efforts into a paragon of fitness.

If current statistics on physical activity are any indication, you are probably doing something, but not enough, to optimize your health. Center for Disease Control (CDC) statistics show that 26.2 percent of Americans met current exercise recommendations in 2001; 46.2 percent did some, but not enough exercise; and 27.6 percent were physically inactive. The National Center for Health Statistics reported that same year that seven out of ten adults did not exercise and that four in ten were completely physically inactive. These numbers have held since 1997, despite a huge amount of media coverage of the dire consequences of being sedentary.

CURRENT GOVERNMENT GUIDELINES

In 2002, the Institute of Medicine (IOM), an independent advisory agency that reports on health issues to the government, released an eight-hundred-page report on the current state of Americans' weight and what should be done about it. It concluded that Americans need to do more and better. They should engage in at least sixty minutes of exercise every day, not the thirty to sixty minutes three to five times a week previously recommended, and they need to pay more attention to the *intensity* of their workouts (more on this later).

I was pleased with these recommendations, as government agencies commonly offer less-than-optimal guidelines because they seem more within reach of the average person. The agencies have not told us to eat whole foods or eat organic or eat vegetables at every meal because of the fear that most people will reject the advice altogether because it seems too difficult to follow.

In so doing, the government misinforms the public, allowing people to think that by doing less than the optimum, they are significantly improving their health. While small changes are better than no changes, big changes are best. Americans are in inexcusably lousy shape and need to face the facts: a half hour of mild to moderate activity three times a week is not going to take off their excess pounds or protect them against chronic diseases.

Our ancestors were physically active throughout their day—lifting, carrying, pushing, and pulling. We're designed to be active. Think of how people lived as recently as one hundred years ago. In 1906, most Americans lived in rural, agrarian environments and spent most of their waking hours engaging in some kind of physical activity. Just preparing a meal was labor-intensive, as people had to harvest crops, slaughter animals, walk to markets, and prepare and cook dishes the old-fashioned way. Today we can easily consume many times the calories we did then, investing little time or effort. In those days you had to burn calories to consume calories, but now you can just bark orders at a fast-food drive-in-window or push a button on your microwave oven.

ADD MORE ACTIVITY TO EACH DAY

Homo sapiens has been around for nearly two hundred thousand years, but until just yesterday, evolutionarily speaking, we were all physically active and ate only natural foods. Thinking that our bodies and minds will not revolt against today's sedentary lifestyles and poor eating is naive at best; at worst, deadly.

Take every opportunity to add physical activity to your life. You can do little things to improve your fitness every day. A few tips:

- When you sit down in or get up from a chair, do not use your hands to push yourself up or lower yourself. Sit and stand ten times, slowly, inhaling as you sit and exhaling as you stand.
- Whenever possible, sit on the floor or, if you're outdoors, on the ground. This will keep your joints flexible. Try squatting too, sitting all the way down on your heels like people in third-world countries who don't have chairs everywhere they go. Japanese women squat a lot more than American women, and they have a lot less osteoporosis and arthritis. Use it or lose it!
- Climb stairs instead of riding the elevator. And when you climb, do so in a slow and focused manner. Take more than one step at a time if you can, holding your body erect with your head directly above your spine, eyes forward, chin tucked down toward your chest.
- Anytime you're waiting in line or standing around, do a little balance training. Stand on one foot with your other foot off the floor. Feel the leg you're standing on stretching tall and straight. Keep your hips level. Place your leg in front of you, to the side, then to the back. Repeat with your other leg. You can also strengthen your calves by doing heel raises.
- Even if you're sitting down, watching TV, talking on the phone, or working on your computer, you can still get a little exercise. Work your abdominal muscles: Start by sitting straight and tall, right on top of your "sitbones" (the two bottom points of the pelvis), then

pull your abdominal muscles in toward your spine—imagine you are pushing your belly button all the way back to your spine. Exhale as you do this. You'll slouch a bit and your lower back will round. Then as you release your abs, sit up straight on your sitbones again.

Don't limit your workout regimen to the indoors. Movement is an important part of interacting with our surroundings and fully sensing our environment. We spend so much time cloistered in cars, offices, gyms, or home entertainment centers, inundated by noise, electrical and electromagnetic energies, and other products of civilization. Going outside and moving your body provides a needed balance for all this chaotic modernity.

The new field of ecopsychology has shown that exposure to nature increases human health and happiness. A full Age Optimization program requires that you spend time in nature.

IF YOU ARE OVERWEIGHT OR VERY UNFIT

Keep in mind that no matter how many years you've been alive, a comprehensive physical training program will make a difference in your health and your appearance—whether you're 28 or 98. But if you have been letting yourself go for a long time, you will have to do forty-five to ninety minutes of moderate cardiovascular training at least five times a week and some weight training to get into shape. If you need a little extra motivation or instruction, buy sessions with a personal trainer.

THE SPIRITUAL BENEFITS OF EXERCISE

In my practice, I hear people making excuse after excuse as to why they don't exercise: they're just too busy, they don't like going to the gym, they're just not motivated to stick with it, they've exercised before but haven't seen any changes . . . so why bother?

Weight loss and physical health aside, moving the body helps us connect with the soul—if we let it. Going to a gym with fluorescent lights and booming rock music and exercising on a machine surrounded by mirrors isn't likely to be a soulful experience. Neither is "going for the burn" or exercising only because we hate our bodies the way they are and want to change them.

When we exercise with awareness, we can enjoy moving, sweating, breathing hard, and stretching, even when they cause some discomfort.

Two kinds of awareness can support our commitment to regular exercise. The first is an interior awareness, where we remain in the present and allow ourselves to experience the body sensations, thoughts, and feelings we are having. If you are exercising and it doesn't feel very good, your self-talk might persuade you to quit long before you derive any benefits. Or you might be doing an exercise that is truly injurious to your body, but because you're tuned out, you keep pushing yourself until you're injured and then you can't exercise.

The second kind of awareness is the knowledge of how exactly exercise benefits your body, both in the short term and the long term.

Exercises for Your Unmentionables: Kegels

Men and women can both lose tone in the muscles of the genital and urinary tracts as they age, which can contribute to urinary incontinence and loss of pleasure during sex. Doing Kegel exercises is a great way to stave off this aspect of the aging process. Consciously toning the muscles in the genitourinary tract can help both men and women improve their continence and sexual responsiveness throughout their lifetimes.

Simply contract the muscles you use to "hold it in" when you have to urinate. Hold the contraction for a few seconds, then release. You can do Kegels several times a day. Try them while you watch TV or drive your car. Include them in your exercise routine. Be consistent; as with any muscle, it's use it or lose it.

EXERCISE LITERACY: KNOW HOW EXERCISE AFFECTS YOUR BODY

Let's look at some of the changes that occur in your body during endurance exercise (also known as aerobic exercise), such as walking, swimming, jogging, cycling, or other full-body activity that increases your heart and respiratory rates and makes you sweat.

When you jog, your cardiac output—the amount of blood your heart pumps in a given time—can rise by a factor of four, from five liters a minute to twenty. Heart rate can increase threefold, and the volume pumped with each heartbeat rises by about 20 milliliters per beat. Blood pressure doesn't rise very much because the blood vessels expand to take on the extra flow. Working muscles take more oxygen from the bloodstream, which leaves less oxygen for areas of the body not involved in exercise, such as the digestive tract. (This is why your mother always told you to rest for a while after eating because exercise slows digestion and can cause gastrointestinal distress.) The blood supply to the brain remains the same while blood flow to the spinal cord rises slightly during an aerobic workout.

Hemoglobin carries oxygen in the bloodstream and releases it to the tissues that need it. As body temperature rises, oxygen increasingly dissociates from hemoglobin, drenching the working muscles with the oxygen they need to burn the carbohydrates and fats they use as fuel.

Skin becomes flushed as skin blood vessels expand, bringing blood close to the body's surface to dissipate heat. The joints, which are filled with lubricating fluid, become warm and pliable, as do the ligaments that connect bones to bones and the tendons that connect muscles to bones. Increased blood flow throughout the body flushes wastes and toxins and rejuvenates the tissues, a process like a dirty sponge being wrung out and allowed to expand again in a bucket of clean water. Levels of natural opiates called endorphins rise, and you start to feel a little buzz from the combination of these endorphins with increased levels of adrenaline and cortisol. This is the "runner's high."

Muscle tissue can only do three things: it can contract, become locked into a state of contraction, or relax. Still, the interplay of the various muscles and the ways in which their interplay moves the skeleton give human beings a versatility of movement and expression unrivalled by any other species. Workouts provide us with a daily opportunity to focus on and be thankful for our bodies' many wondrous capabilities. Truly, the workings of the human musculoskeletal and respiratory systems are marvels of natural engineering that deserve enormous appreciation, even awe.

The ideal workout involves both aerobic exercise (like walking, swimming, basketball, tennis, soccer, running, dancing, climbing, and rowing) and strength training exercise (weightlifting and other types of resistance training). Stretching should be involved too. Shoot for at least four or five workouts weekly; or even better, work out every day.

INTENSITY

The level of effort you put forth during exercise is called intensity. Probably the most common mistake made by novices is that they exercise at either too low or too high an intensity.

When your intensity is too low, you get little benefit from your workout. If you just stroll around the block a few times and never feel out of breath or warm, you are working at too low an intensity. It's better than doing nothing . . . but let's try to optimize your workout time.

If your intensity is too high, you run the risk of doing damage to muscles and joints. You become exhausted quickly, and you don't feel good. Your fight-or-flight response can end up triggered. Too high an intensity can produce an excess of free radicals, resulting in oxidative damage to your body. If you overwork yourself day after day, you will end up with an injury, a compromised immune system, or something worse. Going "over the top" causes your body to conserve fat and burn stored carbohydrates because fats cannot be burned fast enough to provide needed energy for an intense workout.

Unless you are already at a high level of fitness, your intensity should be moderate. What does this mean? When you exercise at a moderate intensity, you will feel exhilarated, not exhausted; pumped-up, not deflated. You will breathe heavily, but you will still be able to carry on a conversation. You will perspire, but your clothes will not be completely drenched with sweat. If you are already fit, you can push the boundaries of intensity with *interval training*: high-intensity intervals alternating with rest or low-intensity intervals. For example, you might run a lap on the local track then walk a lap, and so on.

The intensity of your workout affects your metabolic rate both during and after exercise. When you find that happy middle ground and exercise at a moderate intensity, your body will continue to burn calories at a higher rate than when you are at rest. And this process can continue for a few hours to a whole day. Interval training will boost your post-exercise metabolic rate more than a moderate workout.

MEASURING HEART RATE

The intensity of your exercise is reflected by your heart rate. As you grow fitter, your heart rate falls in response to the same workout, so you have to continue to increase your intensity to continue to benefit from your workout. Let's say, for example, that after walking at 3.5 mph for a couple of weeks, you find that your heart rate no longer rises while you are walking. But once you increase your pace or take a more demanding walk (like walking uphill at the same speed), you will find your heart rate increases to its optimal rate once again.

Invest in a heart rate monitor, or do it the old-fashioned way—with palpation and a watch with a second hand. You can measure heart rate at your wrist or at your carotid artery (gently press two fingertips into the indentation between the thick neck tendons and the jawline). If you cannot find your heartbeat at either of these locations, try placing your hand over your heart.

If you take beta blockers to lower your blood pressure, be aware that your intensity might not be accurately reflected by your heart rate. These drugs suppress the heart rate and blood pressure increase that naturally occur with exercise.

How to Calculate Your Ideal Heart Rate

Applied kinesiologist and chiropractor Dr. Philip Maffetone has developed a variation on the traditional heart rate formula. It's a more versatile formula that takes age, illness, and injury into account. Here's a sample computation for a woman who is sixty-three years old:

1. Subtract your age from 180.
    189 minus 63 equals 126.

2. If you have or are recovering from a major illness or are taking a medication, subtract 10 from 180 minus your age.
None of the above applies to our subject, so we subtract 0 from 126 here.
3. If you have not exercised before or have not exercised in the recent past due to injury or illness, subtract 5.
Our subject recently pulled a hamstring and was sidelined for a week. 126 minus 5 equals 121.
4. If you have been exercising for more than two years without injury and have been getting progressively fitter, add 5.
Or if she hadn't had that injury, we would have added 5 to 126, equaling 131.

The result is your maximum aerobic heart rate, the rate you should attempt to maintain (slightly below is okay also) to derive the best fat-burning and aerobic conditioning benefits.

Divide the result of the formula by six and you will have a ten-second count. Periodically during your workout, check your heart rate for ten seconds and adjust your intensity accordingly. But keep moving, as your heart rate drops quickly when you stop.

Dr. Maffetone points out that his formula works best for people between the ages of sixteen and sixty-five. Those over sixty-five can obtain a misleadingly low figure with this formula. If you are over sixty-five, I suggest you speak with a professional trainer or physical therapist to find out your ideal aerobic heart rate. If you're over sixty-five and clearly healthy and fit, you have no reason to lower your optimal workout heart rate to below what it would be if you were still sixty-five. To be on the safe side, you can use the traditional formula: 220 minus your age (your age-predicted maximum heart rate) times .60 (60 percent of your maximum) and times .80 (80 percent of your maximum). You can work toward the top of the range if you are fit and healthy or keep to the bottom if you are not.

If at all possible, do weight-bearing aerobic exercise. It's better for strengthening bones and muscles than non-weight-bearing exercises such as swimming and stationary cycling. With weight-bearing exercise, the more you weigh, the more energy (calories) you will expend during your workout. Try something adventurous. Sign up for a martial art or a dance class. Try a new kind of aerobic exercise class at the gym. Take up rock climbing or cross-country skiing. Train to walk a half marathon. Let exercise be a chance to learn something new, to expand your horizons.

STRENGTH TRAINING

Although the two types of exercise—aerobic and strength training—are often considered separate entities, they are really just two points along the exercise continuum. When you strength-train properly, you will gain aerobic benefits. Your heart will beat faster, you will breathe heavily, and your body will undergo the changes that result from aerobic work.

Although strength training is good for everyone, it's of paramount importance for aging people. As we age, our muscle mass decreases, and this will happen to some extent no matter what we do. Strength training is the single most valuable tool you have to slow this process. Like weight-bearing aerobic activity, strength training also strengthens bone and connective tissues.

Strength training can be done with free weights or using weight machines. You can also strength-train with elastic bands. Some types of training use the body's own weight as resistance; so-called power yoga involves this kind of strengthening, as does Pilates.

Both yoga and Pilates are highly recommended for sculpting the body, increasing flexibility, improving posture and breathing, and reversing the effects of aging. Yoga is particularly good for relieving stress and moving blood and energy around the body in ways that both cleanse and fortify. The spiritual aspect is central to yoga, and fortunately, your religion (or lack thereof) will not clash with its spiritual teachings. Practicing yoga is a wonderful way to visit the elusive space of inner peace, merging consciousness of the body with enlightenment of the soul.

Yoga teacher Erich Schiffman on the practice of yoga:

> *Yoga is not the dutiful practice of prescribed routines. It is not a paint-by-number practice. It is an ever-new expression of where you are at*

the moment . . . Yoga involves adjusting and readjusting—continuously and with full awareness—so that the ding! feeling [of rightness, of perfect flow, of everything clicking into place] is an ongoing experience . . . This attitude extends out into the way you live your life. Listening for guidance and then doing and being as your deepest feelings prompt you is how you do yoga during the day.

THE UN-EXERCISE: LEARN TO QUIET YOUR MIND

Many of us live in very fast-paced worlds, and our minds are constantly spinning in trying to keep up. We have appointments to keep, bills to pay, children to feed, money to make, social ladders to climb. Many feel that they are on fast-moving treadmills that never stop.

In this age of technology, the amount of information to which we're exposed is growing by leaps and bounds. We are expected to understand this information, use it, and retain it; but typically as soon as we digest one bit, we are bombarded with a dozen more. Our senses and brains were not designed for this kind of onslaught, and it takes a toll. Just trying to filter it to determine which bits are important is an exhausting task.

A body that is sick, in pain, or out of balance doesn't support our ability to think straight, to experience pleasure, to be aware. As we struggle to handle all these challenges, the thing that most often takes a back seat is our health. Learn how to quiet your mind, and you will begin to put your health back where it belongs—at the top of your priority list.

One way to quiet your mind is through meditation. Meditation is about observing your thoughts, not judging them or getting rid of them. During meditation, these thoughts will come, and the trick is to find the space between those thoughts. As you practice quieting your mind, those spaces will become larger and longer.

Stilling the mind helps you to live in the moment. Learning to live in the moment, to enjoy the moment and the reality it contains, is both liberating and empowering. Not only does it help to lessen stress and anxiety, it also teaches us to appreciate what we have, instead of worrying about what we don't have.

If you've never just observed your thoughts without getting embroiled in them or acting upon them, you will find doing so to be difficult at first. It takes practice. It's said that 85 percent of yesterday's thoughts are the same thoughts we have today. Most of these thoughts are about the future, based on what we tell ourselves is our past. Worrying about future events creates stress, anxiety, and depression over things that have not yet happened and probably won't.

Quieting the mind helps us recognize the thoughts we have on a regular basis, the thoughts we think over and over. Thoughts almost always originate in the past, and we project them into an imaginary future. They are usually negative or judgmental; and even though they might no longer be true—or perhaps were never true—they continue, like endlessly looping tapes, to play in our minds. These obsessive thoughts are commonly about things that were said or done to us by significant figures in our lives, or a replaying of certain situations that we experienced.

Meditation can be as simple as spending some time alone in a quiet place, focusing on your breath, and acknowledging your thoughts and feelings. This places you squarely in the present moment. You can expect that your mind will wander, but when it does, acknowledge this and gently refocus your attention on your breathing. That's all there is to it.

This practice will cultivate mindfulness. *Mindfulness* is just another term for living in the moment. As we cultivate mindfulness, we observe who we are; and we become less opinionated, less judgmental. We question our views of the world and our place in it. We become more appreciative of the fullness of each moment. Meditation is the "quality time" you spend with yourself.

Whether you take five minutes or ten or twenty is not that important. You can even meditate for one single minute.

AN EXERCISE PROGRAM FOR LIFE

If you are ready to toss this book out because you're certain that you don't have sixty minutes a day to exercise, hold on a moment. You don't have to exercise for sixty minutes at a stretch. You can split your exercise into shorter periods throughout the day. For example, you can take a twenty-minute walk in the morning, a twenty-minute walk on your lunch break, and then do your strength workout in the evening for your total of sixty minutes.

Do you spend an hour or two watching television every day? How about surfing the Internet? Talking on the phone? You could be exercising. Make exercise a much higher priority. It's that important.

Today is a new day, and you could be putting on your workout clothes instead of beating yourself up or making excuses for not having exercised the day before, the week before, or the month before—or ever.

Also remember that something is better than nothing. Still, this book is about optimization, not doing the bare minimum. "Every day?" you might ask. "Do I have to exercise every day?" No, but it is actually easier to stay with a program if you do it every single day. It becomes part of your routine. One you've established exercise as a daily habit, you miss it if you go a day without doing it. That's when you've made the change from a person who tries to squeeze in exercise whenever possible to someone who has truly integrated physical activity into your life.

CHAPTER TEN

Sexual Healing: Tapping Into the Real Fountain of Youth

Drugs, hormone supplements, and plastic surgery have all changed the world of mature sexuality dramatically. A man can take a capsule of Cialis, a drug in the same class as Viagra, and have sex several times over a couple of days, with enhanced responsiveness and the pleasure of not worrying about whether he'll be able to *perform*. Women can use testosterone and other hormones to maintain their sexual vigor well past menopause too. Both men and women can "have work done" and feel younger and more sexually attractive.

Whether or not such aids are brought into a mature couple's sex life, the latter part of middle age and beyond can be a wonderful time of sexual fulfillment. Changes in hormone levels that naturally occur with aging have the effect of balancing our feminine and masculine energies. Women can become more in touch with their masculine side, and men can learn to enjoy their more passive, softer feminine aspects.

But this period does present its obstacles. For women, loss of libido, painful intercourse, lack of natural lubrication, difficulty reaching orgasm, and self-consciousness about body changes are common. Men can experience a diminishing of sexual desire, difficulty reaching orgasm, and self-consciousness, plus erectile dysfunction, premature ejaculation, and prostate issues. Other adverse factors, especially chronic disease conditions, can cause people to give up on sex completely.

Remaining sexual as we age is not only about "getting off," having good erections, or even about maintaining the strong libido we might once have had. Mature sexuality is not about potency, endurance, or penetration. It's about relating, feeling, and valuing ourselves and our lovers.

RETURNING TO THE BODY

Sexuality can be a source of enlightenment, a release, a great workout, a therapy, a way to connect with a loved one, and a way to awaken body consciousness. Good sex does a lot for the body, the mind, and the soul.

When you read a fairy tale where the heroine and hero ride off into the sunset happily ever after, chances are they will have good sex in their first months together. Whatever they lack in expertise is offset by their sexual energy and physical attraction. But then, often, come children, and the workaday demands of running the kingdom. These things have their own rewards, but the days of hot sex are seemingly over for our fairytale characters. This doesn't have to be the case, not for Cinderella and Prince Charming, or for you.

Arousal and sexual activity do more than make you feel good. Research has demonstrated that they can lead to longer life, bolster resistance against heart disease, alleviate pain, improve immune function, stave off depression, and even guard against cancer:

- A study of 3,500 men found that more frequent intercourse was correlated with greater longevity.
- Men and women who have sex regularly appear to have lowered risk of breast and prostate cancers.
- During peak arousal and orgasm, painkilling signals are sent from brain in the form of endorphins and corticosteroid hormones. A good session of sex can relieve pain from headaches, menstrual cramps, arthritis, and migraine—at least for a few minutes.
- In a study of college students, those who had twice-weekly sex had 30 percent higher levels of a certain antibody than those who did not. (Curiously, those who had sex more than twice a week had

lower levels than those who had no sex at all, so here, as elsewhere, more might not be better.)
- Sex also activates the production of hormones and neurochemicals that reduce anxiety and thus have a calming effect on the body.
- Intercourse burns calories (about 200), and heart rate and blood pressure rise to double their resting levels during orgasm, just as they do during exercise. Formal studies haven't been done yet, but lovemaking "workouts" will almost certainly improve the health of heart and blood vessels.

MAKE LOVE, NOT FEAR

When a man is fearful about sex, he can lose his ability to get or maintain an erection. I see this in my office all the time—men who can't "perform," in part because of their fear of not being able to perform. A woman's sexual anxiety isn't quite so obvious, but this is the number one reason she doesn't have an enjoyable sex life.

If you want to be the best lover you can be, worry less about looking or performing a certain way and focus on finding out what your partner wants and then on giving it to him or her. Communicate as openly as you can about what you want from your partner and help him or her satisfy your desires.

Everybody knows how they want to be loved and what arouses them. Some folks are less willing to openly share what that is, but patience and trust will do the trick with even the most modest partner. Try asking these questions to help him or her convey exactly what he or she wants:

- What kind of environment makes you feel most sexy?
- Where do you want me to touch you?
- How do you want me to talk to you?
- How do you like to be touched?
- How do you want me to kiss you?

If you ask questions like these, and you're careful to respond without judgment or extraneous talk, you will have the precise recipe to produce the desired response in your partner, which will ultimately please both of you.

AGE-RELATED OBSTACLES TO SATISFYING SEX

Many older people have physical problems that come between them and satisfying sex. The astronomical sales of Viagra and other erection-inducing drugs bear witness to one of the most common age-related changes in sexual response. Women over fifty have their own problems, including waning libido, decreased vaginal muscle tone, and decrease in vaginal lubrication. Pharmaceutical companies have been scrambling to find a drug to help older women keep up with their Viagra-popping partners.

Sex after fifty is not the same as sex at twenty-five, beginning with the fact that our bodies stop responding to every kind of stimulus with instantaneous physical desire. We can, however, open ourselves to discovering a deeper, more spiritual kind of lovemaking—one that might or might not involve intercourse and orgasm.

Sexuality after fifty offers the potential for more loving, holding, caressing, spooning, being close, snuggling, and relaxing into sex. Rather than dissipating sexual energy through a quick orgasm, we can cultivate this energy slowly and take the time to more deeply experience the many sensations of lovemaking.

Older people—especially those with medical problems—can require a calm, slow progression to sexual contact and a gentle attitude of acceptance. Be open to experimentation with different positions and different ways of expressing your sexual nature and desires.

At all ages, men and women are turned on by different things. According to Dr. Jennifer Berman, director of the Female Sexual Medicine Center at UCLA, "Women experience desire as a result of context—how they feel about themselves and their partner, how safe they feel, their closeness and their attachment." Men, she says, "tend to be more visually directed and stimulated than women are." Women need to feel good about themselves and safe with their partner; men can look at a pair of breasts and they're ready to go, no matter how they're feeling.

Women, when your man wants to be sexual at a time when you are feeling unsafe and not close, keep this in mind and forgive him, for he can't help that the sight of you turns him on. Men, when you're raring to go and your woman seems aghast that you could even *think* of such a thing at a time like this, forgive her because she may need to feel close to you and not threatened in any way to experience sexual desire for you.

Spend time in relationship. Create a little Garden of Eden and go there on a regular basis. Don't expect lovemaking to arise spontaneously every time. If it does, great; but if it doesn't, set aside regular times for it. This doesn't mean that you will necessarily *have* sex; it just means being together in a quiet, intimate way.

Create a sanctuary for lovemaking. It can be your bedroom, but rather than thinking of your bedroom as a place to watch TV or read before falling asleep, think of it as a place where you and your partner can connect in the deepest of ways. Decorate it with colors and objects that give you aesthetic and sensual pleasure. Keep a stereo nearby, and perhaps a library of erotica. Keep a nice-looking secret "toolbox" with any aids you require: lubricants, massage oils, feathers, or whatever else you like to use to make intimacy more exciting.

Also maintain your hygiene and grooming. All too often as people age, they allow themselves to become unkempt—especially if they have been with the same partner for a long time.

Thich Nhat Hanh talks about the modesty and respect that is traditionally observed in Vietnamese marriages: couples don't undress in front of one another unless intimate activity is going to occur. This is a bit extreme, but it made me realize that many people's sex lives could be enriched with a bit of mystery, a bit of modesty, and the idea that you groom and dress to please your mate.

THE FEELING FUNCTION IN SEXUALITY

Most of us become separated from our feelings during childhood. Our desire to be loved by our parents and to please them became more important than feeling our own feelings. We learned to act in ways that got us the attention and approval we craved. But as we became progressively more disconnected from our feelings, we also got disconnected from our sexuality. This is especially true for boys, who are often criticized or ridiculed by parents and peers if they appeared too sensitive or shy.

Later on, when we were allowed to be overtly sexual, we probably did so according to formulas and ideas that we learned from the media or friends. Sexual experiences can be fraught with fear. At worst, such experiences can seem hollow, devoid of any genuine feelings of desire, safety, and adequacy.

Recovering the sexual feeling function is not easy, but it's a key element of optimizing both sexual life and health. To do so, you must listen to your feelings and acknowledge them often.

SPENDING TIME TOGETHER: THE FOUNDATION OF GREAT SEX

Make an agreement with your partner that once a week, you will meet in your sacred place for some intimate time together. Take at least one hour, preferably two or three. Unplug the telephone, eliminate other distractions, and make sure you will not be interrupted.

Then sit or lie together and experience the energy that flows within and between you. Snuggle. Spoon. Kiss. Play. Laugh. Massage one another. Relax. (Don't fall asleep, though—if it's a nap you need, you do that first, then spend your time together when you are rested.) If you become aroused, do what comes naturally. If you end up having an orgasm, good for you, but again remember that orgasm is not the point. The point is being together and participating in the closeness, however it is expressed.

This is the time to share with your partner exactly what you want. Try dedicating one whole session to nothing but pleasing your partner; then for the next session have your partner reciprocate.

MEN'S SEXUAL DIFFICULTIES AND TREATMENTS

Erectile dysfunction—less elegantly known as impotence—is the inability to maintain an erection long enough to engage in successful intercourse.

Perhaps 30 million American men suffer from ED, amounting to more than 12 percent of the population. This is not a big surprise when you consider that so many common chronic ailments can cause impotence, including hypertension, artery disease, diabetes, and depression. Prostate surgery and trauma can also diminish a man's sexual potency. The anxiety that accompanies ED just compounds the problem.

The standard therapies for erectile dysfunction are drugs that enhance blood flow into the penis upon stimulation. Viagra (sildenafil) and Levitra (vardenafil) are two common ones used for this purpose.

Both of these drugs are known to increase the likelihood of heart attack in men who have preexisting heart disease. These men are more likely to have occluded arteries to the penis. If the vessels to the heart are unhealthy, chances are, these vessels are too. This kind of occlusion is a major cause of erectile dysfunction, and no doubt many men who take these drugs have undiagnosed heart disease. How ironic that ED sufferers with clogged arteries shouldn't take Viagra or Levitra because of the dangers they pose. Any man who wants to use these medications should have a physical first, to ensure that their hearts are in decent shape. Don't try to get a prescription for these drugs without being thoroughly evaluated by a physician! They are not risk free, and you need to be certain they will be safe for you.

Other approaches include vacuum devices (which fit over the penis and use suction to pull blood into it), elastic bands (the erection is maintained with an elastic band at the base of the penis), penile prostheses (surgical implantation of inflatable balloons that are pumped up to create an erection).

Prostaglandins are also used, both intraurethral (pellets containing a prostaglandin drug inserted into the urethra, where the drug is absorbed and produces an erection) and injected. These injections are not painful, as they are done with a tiny, small-gauge needle; and they produce a hard erection that lasts thirty to forty-five minutes. Use of prostaglandins precludes risky surgery, and it's less cumbersome than vacuum devices. Still, in some men, the drug causes pain; and some develop scar tissue from the injections. Consult with a urologist as to which of these therapies would be best if you cannot use Viagra or Levitra.

Over-the-counter vitamin B6 supplements can increase the duration of erections. Minerals like calcium, magnesium, potassium, chromium, and selenium also promote better erectile function in men, with zinc perhaps being the most important for male sexual health and libido.

When I evaluate a man for erectile dysfunction, I consider a lot more than just his physiology. I ask him questions about his feelings, about his childhood, about his relationships. I try to ascertain whether he is in touch with his feeling function, the extent of his awareness of his inner emotional state. And I assess his connection with his soul.

Men are taught to suppress their emotions, to always be "in control," to never admit vulnerability. They are taught to pretend, and then to pretend that they are not pretending—to play roles rather than be themselves. Once their desire and ability to keep an erection fade, many men find few rewards for being sexual. They can blame the women in their lives for their lack of intimacy instead of taking an honest look at their own emotions.

Men must open up to their feeling selves if they are to enjoy the fruits of mature sexuality.

WOMEN'S SEXUAL DIFFICULTIES AND TREATMENTS

Women who suffer from vaginal dryness or atrophy should see significant improvement with estrogen and progesterone replacement therapies. In the case of vaginal dryness, women can choose from a wide variety of sexual lubricants.

Testosterone replacement often works wonders in women who lack libido.

If you're an older woman, you should definitely practice Kegel exercises. Contract the muscles of your vagina as though you were stopping and starting the flow of urine. Start out with ten or twenty reps two to three times a day and increase to fifty to one hundred. Get in the habit of doing your Kegels while you sit in traffic, or stand in line, or watch TV. This is the best way to firm and strengthen the vaginal walls, and it should also help to control stress incontinence—the escape of urine during laughter, sneezing, or coughing.

IF YOU ARE NOT IN A RELATIONSHIP

Keeping in mind the advice given in this chapter and the one on relationships will help you open you up to the best kind of relationship. If you wish to enjoy your sexuality but don't have a partner, try pleasuring yourself in ways you would want a partner to pleasure you. Treat this practice as you would treat intimate time with a lover. Spend time in your sacred space and see what happens.

Those who are not regularly touched, caressed, and held by an intimate partner should make a point of having a massage at least once a week. What this kind of touch lacks in intimacy is offset by the skill of the massage therapist. Have a dialogue with the therapist to make sure you are getting exactly what you need.

Don't be afraid to touch your children and grandchildren more. Even if you have never been a "touchy-feely" kind of person, you'll find they will appreciate this kind of attention. If you feel awkward about this, you can say something to them like "I hope it's all right with you if I touch you more often because I realize that I need more loving touch in my life."

In this day and age, loving touch is often looked upon with suspicion at best, perhaps as inappropriate, and predation at worst. This is tragic, and ironic, because sexual predators were likely not held enough as babies, touched lovingly as children, and probably had impoverished sex and love lives. The answer to the problem of sexual predation is not less touch, nor fear of touch, but more touch—touch from the soul.

EPILOGUE

Just the Beginning

WITH AGE OPTIMIZATION, we maintain a clear mind and a healthy body so we can give our souls the chance to express who we really are, to clarify our goals, to realize our dreams, and to complete the arc of our growth. We extend the lifespan not only to extend our enjoyment of this world, but also to give ourselves the opportunity to transcend our old consciousness and move into a new one. By doing so, we can be part of the solution to the mounting problems the world faces, instead of adding to the burden.

You've learned to optimize the vessel in which you travel through this lifetime. You know that in order to optimize your age, you need to:

- know what foods do in your body and which ones promote your health, and translate this knowledge into wise daily food choices.
- move your body in a mindful and intentional manner on a regular basis.
- make informed choices (informed, when appropriate, by the results of laboratory testing) about whether you will take nutritional supplements and use bio-identical hormones.
- be able to listen—really listen—and acknowledge what you yourself and others are feeling, and to balance feeling and thought.
- let go of what you believe and what you think you know and allow your feelings to be heard.
- be forgiving, accepting and of service.
- find and employ effective methods for reducing the ill effects of stress on your mind, body, and soul.
- laugh at yourself on a regular basis!

- maintain a reasonable sensual life and experience sensual enjoyment of your world and of your partner (if you have one).

Now that you have all this knowledge, stop making feeble attempts to get your health on track. Be willing to do whatever it takes to optimize your health, and don't wait to start until you're already sick. Be proactive. The sooner you begin, the greater your life span as a healthy, high-energy elder is likely to be. With this in place, you are ready to do the work of shifting and elevating your consciousness.

What, then, are the steps one must take to shift one's consciousness? This has been a lifelong subject of great interest to me. When I'm not practicing medicine or spending time with family and friends, I study this topic. In the companion book to this one, I hope to serve as a guide for you as I share what I have learned about moving into a new consciousness in a vibrant, well-cared-for body. In this regard, this Epilogue is not the end, but the beginning of the journey.

The earliest humans existed at a level of consciousness that was mostly about instinct and survival. Choices were made for the simple purpose of staying alive. Primitive tribal humans and medieval humans existed at a slightly higher level of consciousness, where they developed a dualistic view of the world: other humans were seen as friends or foes. In today's world, many human beings remain stuck in this level of consciousness. We must be right, others must be wrong; those who don't share our beliefs are our enemies; you're either with us or against us. This state creates war, strife, opposition between the sexes, genocide, and other kinds of unnecessary and tragic conflict. This is a reactionary state—a higher level of awareness than instinct, but still a low level of awareness.

The next level of consciousness is beautifully illustrated by Shakespeare's Hamlet. The play's eponymous character embodies the state of modern man: uncertain, totally confused, equivocating, disorderly. He has instincts and drives, but cannot get himself to act upon them until it's too late. A less reactionary state, certainly, and more evolved than the state that precedes it; but as we can see from the disasters created by modern politicians, CEOs, and others in power, people in this state are ill-equipped to solve the world's problems. They're too mired in ego concerns, which make decisive choice difficult and wisdom hard to achieve.

The ego is a necessary part of the soul's journey—the part of the human being that enables it to become part of a family, a village, a society, a culture. It gives identity and helps us to choose our roles in life. The evolution to the next stage of consciousness means becoming clear that you are not the ego. You are not the indecisive voice that prattles endlessly in your head. Your true self is the self that can see the ego doing its thing, but that does not identify with that ego.

If this realization does not come, we remain out of balance, unable to act with purpose or direction. We are unable to make clear and wise choices because we are disconnected from our souls, existing instead in the egoic mind and all its chatter, its competitiveness, its identification with objects and power. Modern humankind feels alienated from life's purpose and meaning, and so it becomes susceptible to a herd mentality. At this level of consciousness, we are intensely vulnerable to influences that do not work towards the good of all, or even of ourselves.

To move upward from this level of consciousness and those beneath it, we must connect with that which gives us meaning: the feeling self, the soul. When enough people reach this fourth level of consciousness, we can grow into a more loving, forgiving, accepting, and compassionate species. When enough human beings step into this heightened level of consciousness, a sort of critical mass will have accrued, and there will be renewed hope for the present and future of our beleaguered species.

The doubling of the human life span in only 150 years has not happened by accident. Human beings have not evolved significantly for the last 50,000 years—but now, changes are beginning to happen. We're living much longer. We must be grateful for this extra time, preserve the vessel of the body as best we can, and become a force for heightening consciousness and preserving this miraculous human race. This is what the universe is asking of us.

Those who make this shift might be known as a "4-D" person: a person of four dimensions. This is a person who has found his or her soul, who has meaning and purpose in life and whose egoic life is aligned with that soul center. Masculine and feminine can reconnect and live in balance, as can the energies of ego and soul. This process will be the focus of my future books.

Why is the universe granting you this extra time? How will you become part of the critical mass of individuals who are evolving in consciousness? What part will you play in the new human story, where we will see beyond conflict, competition and confusion? Discover why you have been called.

The reason you get to live longer in a healthy body is that you may partake of the journey of your true life. You have an opportunity to take the hero's journey. The journey is difficult. It involves suffering and takes time. You have to dwell in the belly of the whale—to experience the dark night of the soul. The rewards are enormous: in transcending lower levels of consciousness, you reconnect with the Divine.

> I am not I.
>   I am this one
> Walking beside me whom I do not see.
> Whom at times I manage to visit,
> And at other times I forget.
> The one who remains silent when I talk,
> The one who forgives, sweet, when I hate,
> The one who takes a walk when I am indoors,
> The one who will remain standing when I die.

by Juan Ramon Jimenez
(Translated by Robert Bly)

RESOURCES

The **Cenegenics Medical Institute** is worth investigating if you are serious about embarking on a complete Age Optimization program. Its highly qualified staff of physicians can design a program just for you. The company's Web site has much valuable, up-to-date information: http://www.cenegenics.com/. The Institute also offers lab testing by mail.

The **American Academy of Anti-Aging Medicine** (A4M) is a good resource for finding a physician in your area who can help you with bio-identical hormone therapy and other age-optimizing practices described in this book. Visit its Web site at http://www.worldhealth.net/.

Another resource for finding a physician and collecting information on nutrition is the **Institute for Functional Medicine,** at http://www.functionalmedicine.org/.

Women who want more info on natural hormone replacement can visit the Official Web site of John R. Lee, M.D. at *http://www.johnleemd.com/*, or Virginia Hopkins' site at *www.hopkinstestkits.com*.

Women can buy salivary hormone tests at David Zava's ZRT Laboratory Web site, at *http://www.salivatest.com/*.

Barry Sears's books have been indispensable resources for me. If you wish to read more on the science behind my eating recommendations, try his books. My favorites are *Enter the Zone*, with Bill Lawren, the original smash bestseller that first brought eicosanoid balance and the dangers of high insulin to the public's attention; and then *The Omega Rx Zone,* which focuses on the benefits of pharmaceutical-grade fish oil. I also recommend that you check out the Sears Web site. You can purchase pharmaceutical-grade fish oil and lab tests here, in addition to his books: DrSears.com (http://www.drsears.com/).

Pharmaceutical-grade supplements can also be purchased through LifeExtension, at *http://www.lef.org/*.

LAB TESTING

STANDARD TESTS

TABLE 2 LISTS standard laboratory test levels for hormones. Tests should be performed every six to seven weeks to keep levels within ideal ranges. Periodic dose adjustment is often needed.

HORMONE	RANGE
Cortisol	8-18 mg/dL
DHEA	350-500 mcg/dL
Estradiol (men)	< 40 pg/ml
Estradiol (women)	80-100 pg/ml
Insulin-like growth factor 1 (marker of growth hormone activity)	250-320 ng/ml
Progesterone (women)	1-3 ng/ml
Prostate Specific Antigen (PSA, men)	0-4 mcg/L
Testosterone (men)	700-900 ng/dL (total) 130-190 ng/dL (free)
Testosterone (women)	50-70 ng/dL (total) 7-8.5 pg/mL (free)
Thyroid stimulating hormone (TSH)	0.4-5.5

Table 2 Standard lab test hormone levels

Table 3 notes heart disease risk factors.

HORMONE	RANGE
Total cholesterol	0-200 mg/dL
HDL cholesterol	50-200 mg/dL
LDL cholesterol	0-100 mg/dL
Coronary risk ratio (HDL/LDL)	1-3.5
VLDL cholesterol	4-40 mg/dL
Triglycerides	0-100 mg/dL
Homocysteine	5.4-11.4 umol/L
C-Reactive Protein	0-1.0 mg/dL
Blood Pressure	<= 120/80

Table 3 Heart disease risk factors

NEW TESTS

Following are new kinds of blood tests, which better predict your risk of heart disease, especially if you're a person who does not seem to be at risk. They measure lipid subfractions and proteins that attach to lipids. You might have to ask specifically for these tests; I recommend you do so.

Lp(a): Lipoprotein (a) is an LDL particle attached to an abnormal protein; A high Lp(a) increases the risk of coronary artery disease threefold.

HDL subclassification: Helps doctors to determine which therapy would be best to increase HDL.

Apolipoprotein A-1: One of several proteins that attach to HDL particles and can help to predict risk of heart disease.

Apolipoprotein E: This test distinguishes between normal and abnormal forms of this protein. Some forms signify greater likelihood of having high blood lipids and can predict heart disease risk independent of other factors.

Apolipoprotein B-100: Gives a more detailed look at LDL concentrations than standard cholesterol tests.

OTHER RECOMMENDED TESTS

See if you can't get yourself tested for the following once per year:

- Aerobic exercise capacity
- Body fat/waist-to-hip ratio
- Bone density
- Cognitive functioning and mood
- Dementia
- Libido and sexual performance
- Muscular strength
- Quality of life
- Sleep quality

Be sure to undergo all recommended cancer screenings for your age group. Cancers of the colon, skin, testicles, prostate, and breast can all be detected early enough to make a cure almost guaranteed.

By tracking all these health and fitness indicators, you will be able to detect problems long before they threaten your overall well-being.

GLYCEMIC FOOD INDEX GUIDE

LOW-GLYCEMIC VEGETABLES: EAT OFTEN

- Asparagus
- Broccoli
- Cabbage
- Cauliflower
- Celery
- Cucumber
- Green beans
- Leafy greens (spinach, collards, kale, chard, endive)
- Onion
- Radish
- Summer squash
- Tomato
- Zucchini

HIGH-GLYCEMIC VEGETABLES: AVOID

- Beet
- Carrot
- Corn
- Parsnip
- Pumpkin
- Tubers and roots (including potatoes; occasional yams or sweet potatoes are okay)
- Winter squash

LOW-GLYCEMIC FRUITS: EAT OFTEN

- Apple
- Berries

- Cherry
- Dried apricot
- Grapefruit
- Orange
- Peach
- Pear
- Plum

HIGH-GLYCEMIC FRUITS: AVOID

- Banana
- Cantaloupe
- Mango
- Papaya
- Pineapple
- Raisins
- Watermelon

GENERAL EATING TIPS BASED ON GLYCEMIC INDEX GUIDELINES

Base each meal around a lean protein source. Try skinless chicken or turkey, eggs, ocean fish, lamb, lean beef (no more than five times a week), legumes, shellfish (once a week max), tuna or chicken salad (use canola mayonnaise in small amounts).

Dairy should be organic, low-fat. Use butter for cooking. Have small servings of cheeses fewer than five times weekly. Low-fat cottage cheese and cream cheese are fine, and unsweetened plain yogurt can be mixed with fresh berries or cherries.

Ensure that you're getting plenty of good fats. Use organic, cold or expeller-pressed oils. Eat avocado, raw almonds, raw cashews, raw macadamia nuts, salmon, sardines, tuna, canola oil (try Newman's Own dressings, which are made with canola), and olive oil, all in moderation.

Avoid white bread or flour products made with hydrogenated oils. Eat starches three or fewer times a week, in small amounts. One-hundred-percent rye, pumpernickel, whole grain pita, and protein-enriched breads are good choices. Eat steel-cut oatmeal or rolled oats if you like oatmeal. Try pastas made with flour ground from legumes, artichokes, spinach, or soy; stick with brown and wild rices.

REFERENCES

A

Acitelli LK, Antonucci TC, "Gender differences in the link between marital support and satisfaction in older couples," *J Pers Soc Psychol* 1994 Oct;67(4):688-98.

Aisen PS, et al., "A pilot study of vitamins to lower plasma homocysteine levels in Alzheimer's disease," *Am J Geriatr Psychiatry* 2003 Mar-Apr;11(2):246-9.

Alfthan G, Aro A, Gey KF, "Plasma homocysteine and cardiovascular disease mortality," *Lancet* 1997 349: 397.

Amato G, Carella C, Fazio S et al., "Body Composition, Bone Metabolism, and Heart Structure and Function in Growth Hormone(GH)-Deficient Adults Before and After GH Replacement Therapy at Low Doses," *Journal of Clinical Endocrinology and Metabolism* 1993:77:1671-1676.

Ames BN (2001) DNA damage from micronutrient deficiencies is likely to be a major cause of cancer. *Mutat Res* 475(1-2):7-20.

Amory JK, et al, "Exogenous testosterone or testosterone with finasteride increases bone mineral density in older men with low serum testosterone," *J Clin Endocrinol Metab* 2004 Feb;89(2):503-10.

Antonucci TC, Fuhrer R, Dartigues JF, "Social relations and depressive symptomatology in a sample of community-dwelling French older adults," *Psychol Aging* 1997 Mar;12(1):189-95.

Appleton J, "Arginine: clinical potential of a semi-essential amino," *Altern Med Rev* 2002 Dec;7(6):512-22.

Associated Press, "Obesity is going to extremes, study reports," *LA Times*, Tuesday, October 14, 2003:A16.

Attanasio A et al., "Consensus guidelines for the diagnosis and treatment of adults with growth hormone deficiency: Summary statement of the growth hormone research society workshop on adult growth hormone deficiency," *J Clin Endocrinol Metab* 1998;83:379-381.

Auborn KJ, et al., "Indole-3-carbinol is a negative regulator of estrogen," J Nutr. 2003 Jul;133(7 Suppl):2470S-2475S.

B

Bae SC, Kim SJ, Sung MR, "Inadequate antioxidant nutrient intake and altered plasma antioxidant status of rheumatoid arthritis patients," *J Am Coll Nutr* 2003 Aug;22(4):311-5.

Balluz LZ, et al., "Vitamin and mineral supplement use in the US: Results from the 3rd National Health and Nutrition Examination Survey," *Arch Fam Med* 2000;9(3).

Barrett-Connor E, Grady D, "Hormone replacement therapy, heart disease, and other considerations," *Annu Rev Publ Health* 1998;19:55-72.

Bartke A, "Growth hormone and aging," *Endocrine* 1998;8:103-108.

Beck MA, Levander OA, "Host nutritional status and its effect on a viral pathogen," *Biol Trace Elem Res* 2001 Apr;80(1):23-31.

Beck MA et al., "Selenium deficiency increases the pathology of an influenza virus infection," *FASEB J* 2001 Jun;15(8):1481-3.

Betancourt-Albrecht M, Cunningham GR, "Hypogonadism and diabetes," *Int J Impot Res* 2003 Aug;15Suppl4:S14-20.

Bland, Jeffrey, et al., *Clinical Nutrition: A Functional Approach*, The Institute for Functional Medicine, Gig Harbor WA:1999.

Booth GL, Wang EL, with the Canadian Task Force on Preventive Health Care, "Preventive health care, 2000 update: screening and management of hypohomocysteinemia for the prevention of coronary artery disease events," *Canadian Medical Association Journal* 2000;163:21-29.

Brown, David, "Research points to a key Alzheimer's risk factor," *The Washington Post*, Thursday, Feb 14, 2002;A01.

Bosma H, Peter R, Siegrist J, Marmot M, "Two alternative job stress models and the risk of coronary heart disease," *Am J Public Health* 1998 Jan;88(1):68-74.

Brown SL, et al., "Providing social support may be more beneficial than receiving it: results from a prospective study of mortality," *Psychol Sci.* 2003 Jul;14(4):320-7. Berkman LF, Syme SL, "Social networks, host resistance, and mortality: a nine-year follow-up study of Alameda County residents," *Am J Epidemiol* 1979 Feb;109(2):186-204.

Burke BE, et al., "Randomized, double-blind, placebo-controlled trial of coenzyme Q10 in isolated systolic hypertension," *South Med J* 2001 Nov;94(11):1112-7.

Burke BE, Neuenschwander R, Olson RD, "Randomized, double-blind, placebo-controlled trial of coenzyme Q10 in isolated systolic hypertension," *South Med J* 2001 Nov;94(11):1112-7.

C

Carr A, Frei B, "The role of natural antioxidants in preserving the biological activity of endothelium-derived nitric oxide," *Free Radic Biol Med* 2000 Jun 15;28(12):1806-14.

Cape, Coe, and Rossman, eds., *Fundamentals of Geriatric Medicine*, Raven Press, New York: 1983.

Cascieri MA, "The potential for novel anti-inflammatory therapy for coronary artery disease," *Nat Rev Drug Discov* 2002 Feb;1(2):122-30.

Chandraskaren A, et al., "Placebo-controlled trial of indole-3-carbinol in the treatment of CIN," *Gynecol Oncol* 2000 Aug;78(2):123-9.

Chopra D, with David Simon, Grow Younger Live Longer: 10 Steps to Reverse Aging, Harmony Books:2001.

Chromiak JA, Antonio J, "Use of amino acids as growth hormone-releasing agents by athletes," *Nutrition* 2002 Jul-Aug;18(7-8):657-61.

Clarke R, et al, "Folate, vitamin B12, and serum total homocysteine levels in confirmed Alzheimer disease." *Archives of Neurology* 1998 55: 1449-55.

Conis, Elena, "Antioxidants: Have they been hyped?" *LA Times,* Monday, October 27:F1.

Collins P, "Clinical cardiovascular studies of hormone replacement therapy," *Am J Cardiol* 2002 Jul 3;90(1A):30F-34F.

Cook JW, et al, "Homocysteine and arterial disease. Experimental mechanisms," *Vascul Pharmacol* 2002 May;38(5):293-300.

Coppen A, Bailey J, "Enhancement of the antidepressant action of fluoxetine by folic acid: a randomised, placebo controlled trial," *J Affect Disord* 2000 Nov;60(2):121-30.

D

Dandona P, Alijada A, "A rational approach to pathogenesis and therapy of type 2 diabetes mellitus, insulin resistance, inflammation, and atherosclerosis," *Am J Cardiol* 2002 Sep 5;90(5A):27G-33G.

deBruin VM, et al., "Cortisol and dehydroepiandrosterone sulfate plasma levels and their relationship to aging, cognitive function, and dementia," *Brain Cogn* 2002 Nov;50(2):316-23.

Dimitriou T, Maser-Gluth C, Remer T, "Adrenocortical activity in healthy children is associated with fat mass," *Am J Clin Nutr* 2003 Mar;77(3):731-6.

Diaz MN, et al., "Antioxidants and atherosclerotic heart disease," *NEJM* 1997 Aug 7;337(6):408-16.

DiSomma G, et al., "Severe impairment of bone mass and turnover in Cushing's disease: comparison between childhood-onset and adulthood-onset disease," *Clin Endocrinol (Oxf)* 2002 Feb;56(2):153-8.

Doshi SN, et al., "Lowering plasma homocysteine with folic acid in coronary vascular disease: what will the trials tell us?" *Atherosclerosis* 2002 Nov;165(1):1-3.

Dwyer J, unpublished study on vitamin C and arterial thickening, presented at American Heart Association meeting, March 2, 2000, San Diego CA.

E

Ebly EM, et al. Folate status, vascular disease and cognition in elderly Canadians. Age and Ageing 1998 27: 485-491.

Edmonds SE, et al., "Putative analgesic activity of repeated oral doses of vitamin E in the treatment of rheumatoid arthritis. Results of a prospective placebo-controlled double-blind trial," *Ann Rheum Dis* 1997 Nov;56(11):649-55.

Egger T, et al., "Vitamin E (alpha-tocopherol) attenuates cyclo-oxygenase 2 transcription and synthesis in immortalized murine BV-2 microglia," *Biochem J* 2003 Mar;370 (Pt2):459-67.

Engler MM, et al., "Antioxidant vitamins C and E improve endothelial function in children with hyperlipidemia: Endothelial Assessment of Risk for Lipids in Youth (EARLY) Trial," *Circulation* 2003 Sep 2;108(9):1059-63.

Enig, Mary G., Know Your Fats: The Complete Primer for Understanding the Nutrition of Fats, Oils, and Cholesterol, Bethesda Press, Bethesda MD: 2000.

F

Farr SA, et al., "The antioxidants alpha lipoic acid and N-acetylcysteine reverse memory impairment and brain oxidative stress in aged SAMP8 mice," *J Neurochem* 2003 Mar;84(5):1173-83.

Fisher, Helen, "Your Brain In Love," *Time,* January 19, 2004.

Fletcher AE, Breeze E, Shetty PS, "Antioxidant vitamins and mortality in older person: findings from the nutrition add-on study to the Medical research Council trial of assessment and management of older people in the community," *Am J Clin Nutr* 2003 Nov;78(5):999-1010.

Fogerty A, et al., "Dietary vitamin E, IgE concentrations, and atopy," *Lancet* 2000 Nov 4;356(9241):1573-4.

Folkers K, et al., "The activities of coenzyme Q10 and vitamin B6 for immune responses," *Biochem Biophys Res Commun* 1993 May 28;193(1):88-92.

Franchesci C, "Centenarians as a model for healthy aging," *Biochem Soc Trans* 2003;31(457-61).

Frei B, Kim MC, Ames BN, "Ubiquinol-10 is an effective lipid-soluble antioxidant at physiological concentrations," *Proc Natl Acad Sci U S A* 1990 87(12):4879-83.

Fuchs CS, et al., "The influence of folate and multivitamin use on the familial risk of colon cancer in women," *Canc Epid Biom Prev* 2002 Mar;11(3):227-3.

Fujimoto S, et al., "Effects of coenzyme Q10 administration on pulmonary function and exercise performance in patients with chronic lung diseases," *Clin Investig* 1993;71(8 Suppl):S162-6.

Fuke C, Krakorian S, Couris R, "Coenzyme Q10: A review of essential functions and clinical trials," http://www.healingedge.net/briefs_coq10.html

G

Garcia-Estrada J, et al., "An alpha lipoic acid-vitamin E mixture reduces post-embolism lipid peroxidation, cerebral infarction, and neurological deficit in rats," *Neurosci Res* 2003 Oct;47(2):219-24.

Gaynor P, "L-Carnitine Offers Natural Support for Male Fertility," Paula Gaynor, PhD, *Health Supplement Retailer*, Jan 2001, pg. 34.

Goldstat R, et al., "Transdermal testosterone therapy improves well-being, mood, and sexual function in premenopausal women," Jean Hailes Foundation Research Unit, Clayton, Victoria, Australia, amd the Dept of Epidemiology and Preventive Medicine, Monash University, Central and Eastern Clinical School, Prahran, Victoria, Australia.

Granato, Heather, "Coloring consumers' health with carotenoids," *Natural Products Industry Insider,* Nov 2003:36.

Goralska M, et al., "Alpha lipoic acid changes iron uptake and storage in lens epithelial cells," *Exp Eye Res* 2003 Feb;76(2):241-8.

Greenwood-Robinson, Maggie, "Start your fat-burning engine," *Let's Live,* 2001 Dec;30.

H

Hackam DG, et al., "What level of plasma homocyst(e)ine should be treated? Effects of vitamin therapy on progression of carotid atherosclerosis in patients with homocyst(e)ine levels above and below 14 micromol/L," *American Journal of Hypertension* 13:105-100, 2000.

Hajjar IM, et al., "A randomized, double-blind, controlled trial of vitamin C in the management of hypertension and lipids," *Am J Ther* 2002 Jul-Aug;9(4):289-93.

Hajjar RR, Kaiser FE, Morley JE, "Outcomes of long-term testosterone replacement in older hypogonadal males: a retrospective analysis," *J Clin Endocr Metab* 1997 Nov;82(11):3793-6.

Hanioka T, et al., "Effect of topical application of coenzyme Q10 on adult periodontitis," *Mol Aspects Med* 1994;15 Suppl:s241-8.

Hansen IL, et al., Bioenergetics in clinical medicine. IX. Gingival and leucocytic deficiencies of coenzyme Q10 in patients with periodontal disease. Res Commun Chem Pathol Pharmacol. 1976 Aug;14(4):729-38

Hargreaves P, "Ubiquinone: cholesterol's reclusive cousin," *Ann Clin Biochem* 2003 May;40(Pt3):207-18.

Hartmann A, et al., "Vitamin E prevents exercise-induced DNA damage," *Mutat Res* 1995 Apr;346(4):195-202.

Heitzer T, et al., "Endothelial dysfunction, oxidative stress, and risk of cardiovascular events in patients with cardiovascular disease," *Circulation* 2001 Nov 27;104(22):2673-8.

Hendricks, Gay; *Conscious Living: Finding Joy in the Real World*, 2001. HarperSanFrancisco, San Francisco, CA, USA.

Hendricks, Gay, and Hendricks, Kathlyn; *Conscious Loving: The Journey to Co-Commitment*, 1992. Bantam Books, New York, NY, USA.

Hensley K, et al., "New perspectives on vitamin E: gamma-tocopherol aand carboxyeltylhydroxychroman metabolites in biology and medicine," *Free Rad Biol Med* 2004 Jan;36(1):1-15.

Hodgson JM, et al., "Coenzyme Q10 improves blood pressure and glycaemic control: a controlled trial in subjects with type 2 diabetes," *Eur J Clin Nutr* 2002 Nov;56(11):1137-42.

Hoffman, David, B.Sc. (Hons.), M.N.I.M.H., "The Biology of Aging," http://www.healthy.net/scr/article.asp?id=1325

Holmquist C, et al., "Multivitamin supplements are inversely associated with risk of myocardial infarction in women and men—Stockholm Heart Epidemiology Program (SHEEP)," *J Nutr* 2003 Aug;133(8):2650-4.

Hong JH, et al., "Effects of vitamin E on oxidative stress and membrane fluidity in brain of streptozotocin-induced diabetic rats," *Clin Chim Acta* 2004 Feb;340(1-2):107-15.

Hoschl C, Hajek T, "Hippocampal damage mediated by corticosteroids—a neuropsychiatric research challenge," *Eur Arch Psychiatry Clin Neurosci* 2001;251 Suppl 2: II81-8.

House JS, Robbins C, Metzner HL, "The association of social relationships and activities with mortality: prospective evidence from the Tecumseh Community Health Study," *Am J Epidemiol* 1982 Jul;116(1):123-40.

Hu FB, Willett WC, "Optimal diets for prevention of heart disease," *JAMA* 2002 Nov 27;288(20):2569-78.

I

Ingersoll-Dayton B, Antonucci TC, "Reciprocal and nonreciprocal social support: contrasting sides of intimate relationships," *J Gerontol* 988 May;43(3):S65-73.

J

Jacobs E, et al, "Multivitamin use and colorectal cancer incidence in a US cohort: does timing matter?" *Am J Epidemiol* 158;621-28.

James, Jamie, and Weeks, David, *Secrets of the Superyoung: The Scientific Reasons Some People Look 10 Years Younger Than They Really Are—and How You Can, Too*, Villard: 1998.

Julliet P, et al., "Plasma coenzyme Q10 concentrations in breast cancer: prognosis and therapeutic consequences," *Int J Clin Pharmacol Ther* 1998 Sep;36(9):506-9.

Joseph, Stephen L, "Citizen petition regarding trans fat labeling," BanTransFats.com, 2003 May 22.

Juul A, Skakkebaek NE, "Androgens and the ageing male," *Hum Reprod Update* 2002 Sep-Oct;8(5):423-33.

Juul A, Skakkebaek NE, "Androgens and the ageing male," *Hum Reprod Update* 2002 Sep-Oct;8(5):423-33.

K

Kang JH, Shi YM, Zheng RL, "Effects of ascorbic acid on human hepatoma cell proliferation and differentiation," *Zhongguo Yao Li Xue Bao* 1999 Nov;20(11):1019-24.

Kang SS, et al., "Hyperhomocyst(e)inemia as a risk factor for occlusive vascular disease," *Annual Review of Nutrition* 1992;12:279-298.

Katz DL, "Acute effects of oats and vitamin E on endothelial responses to ingested fat," *Am J Prevent Med* 2001;20(2):124-129.

Kimura S, et al., "Docosahexaenoic acid attenuated hypertension and vascular dementia in stroke-prone spontaneously hypertensive rats," *Neurotoxicol Teratol* 2002 Sep-Oct;24(5):683-93.

Klatz, R, DO, MD, *Grow Young With HGH,* New York: Harper Perennial, 1997. Key TJ, et al (Endogenous Hormones Breast Cancer Collaborative Group), "Body mass index, serum sex hormones, and breast cancer risks in postmenopausal women," *Journal of the National Cancer Institute,* 2003 Aug 20;95(16):1218-26.

Krause N, Shaw BA, "Giving social support to others, socioeconomic status, and changes in self-esteem in late life," *J Gerontol B Psychol Sci Soc Sci* 2000 Nov;55(6):S323-33.

Krishnaswamy K, Lakshmi AV, "Role of nutritional supplements in reducing the levels of homocysteine," *J Assoc Physicians India* 2002 May;50 Suppl:36-42.

Kronenberg F, Fugh-Berman A, "Complementary and alternative medicine for menopausal symptoms: a review of randomized, controlled trials," *Ann Intern Med* 2002 Nov 19;137(10):805-13.

Kuller LH, "Hormone therapy and risk of cardiovascular disease: implications of the results of the Women's Health Initiative," *Arterioscler Thromb Vasc Biol* 2003 Jan 1;23(1):11-6.

L

Lampertico M, Comis S, "Italian multicenter study on the efficacy and safety of coenzyme Q10 as adjuvant therapy in heart failure," *Clin Investig* 1993;71:S129-33.

Lee DJ, Markides KS, "Activity and mortality among aged persons over an eight-year period," *J Gerontol* 1990 Jan;45(1):S39-42.

Lee AL, Ogle WO, Sapolsky RM, "Stress and depression: possible links to neuron death in the hippocampus," *Bipolar Disord* 2002 Apr;4(2):117-28.

Lee, John MD, and Virginia Hopkins, *What Your Doctor May Not Tell You About Menopause,* Warner Books, New York, NY:1996.

Lee, John, Jesse Hanley, and Virginia Hopkins, *What Your Doctor May Not Tell You About Premenopause,* Warner Books, New York, NY: 2000.

Leonetti HB, Wilson KJ, Anasti JN, "Topical progesterone cream has an antiproliferative effect on estrogen-stimulated endometrium," *Fertil Steril* 2003 Jan;79(1):221-2.

Lemonick, Michael, "Chemistry of Desire," *Time,* January 19, 2004.

Lincoln KD, Taylor RJ, Chatters LM, "Correlates of emotional support and negative interaction among older Black Americans," *J Gerontol B Psychol Sci Soc Sci* 2003 Jul;58(4):S225-33.

Liu J, Killilea DW, Ames BN (2002) Age-associated mitochondrial oxidative decay: improvement of carnitine acetyltransferase substrate-binding affinity and activity in brain by feeding old rats acetyl-L-carnitine and/or R-alpha-lipoic acid. *Proc Natl Acad Sci U S A* 99(4):1876-81.

Liu G, et al., "Omega 3 but not omega 6 fatty acids inhibit AP-1 activity and cell transformation in JB6 cells," *Proceedings of the National Academy of Sciences* 2001;98(13):7510.

Lockwood K, et al., "Partial and complete regression of breast cancer in patients in relation to dosage of coenzyme Q10," *Biochem Biophys Res Commun* 1994 Mar 30;199(3):1504-8.

Lockwood K, et al., "Progress on therapy of breast cancer with vitamin Q10 and the regression of metastases," *Biochem Biophys Res Commun* 1995 Jul 6;212(1):172-7.

Loralie J, et al., "Hyperhomocyst(e)inemia and the Increased Risk of Venous Thromboembolism," *Archives of Internal Medicine* 2000;160:961-964.

Low AK, et al., "Hormone replacement therapy and coronary heart disease in women: a review of the evidence," *Am J Med Sci* 2002 Oct;324(4):180-4.

M

Marracci GH, et al., "Alpha lipoic acid inhibits T cell migration into the spinal cord and suppresses and treats experimental autoimmune encephalomyelitis," *J Neuroimmunol* 2002 Oct;131(1-2):104-14.

Malinow MR, et al., "Homocyst(e)ine, eating, and cardiovascular diseases: A statement for healthcare professionals from the nutrition committee, American Heart Association," *Circulation* 1999;99:178-182.

Marchioli R, et al., "Antioxidant vitamins and prevention of coronary vascular disease: epidemiological and clinical trial data," *Lipids* 2001;36Suppl:S53-63.

Masaki KH, et al., "Association of vitamin E and C supplement use with cognitive function and dementia in elderly men," *Neurology* 2000 March 28;54:1265-1272.

Maugh, TH II, and Rosie Mestel, "Hormone Therapy's Future Put In Doubt," *LA Times,* Tuesday, March 18, 2003:A1.

Mayne ST, et al., "Nutrient intake and risk of subtypes of esophageal and gastric cancer," *Cancer Epid Biom Prev* 2001 Oct;10(10):1055-62.

McCaddon A, et al., "Total serum homocysteine in senile dementia of Alzheimer type," *International Journal of Geriatric Psychiatry* 1998 13: 235-9.

Mertens A, Holvoet P, "Oxidized HDL and LDL: antagonists in atherothrombosis," *FASEB J* 2001 Oct;15(12):2075-84.

Mintz, Alan MD, lecture titled "Hormonal assessment of the Aging Profile," given at Eastern Virginia Medical School in January, 2002.

Mishra GD, et al., "Childhood and adult dietary vitamin E intake and cardiovascular disease risk factors in mid-life in the 1946 British Birth cohort," *Eur J Clin Nutr* 2003 Nov;57(11):1418-25.

Moss, Ralph W, *Antioxidants Against Cancer*, Equinox Press, Gilroy, CA.

Munkholm H, et al., "Coenzyme Q10 treatment in serious heart failure," *Biofactors* 1999;9(2-4):285-9.

Nelson HD, et al., "Postmenopausal hormone replacement therapy: scientific review," *JAMA* 2002 Aug 21;288(7):872-81.

N

National Center for Health Statistics; "Second National Health and Nutrition Examination Survey (NHANES II) Public-Use Data Files," Hyattsville, MD, USA. http://www.cdc.gov/nchs/products/elec_prods/subject/nhanesii.htm. See this site for other NHANES studies and related research.

No authors listed, Diet Industry is Big Business," CBSNews.com, December 1, 2006; posted at *http://www.cbsnews.com/stories/2006/12/01/eveningnews/main2222867.shtml*, accessed 1-16-08.

No authors listed, "Nutritional Values Decline," *Life Extension*, March 2001:28.

No authors listed, "Testosterone Attacked by the Media," *Life Extension*, Feb 2004.

No authors listed, "The Free Radical Theory of Aging," http://www.thaiwave.com/networkantioxidants/agingtheory.htm

No authors listed, "Can cutting calories increase longevity?"

http://www.infoaging.org/b-cal-home.html

No authors listed, "Resveratrol may increase lifespan," *Natural Products Industry Insider*, September 10, 2003:16. Study published online at *http://www.nature.com/* on August 24, 2003.

No authors listed, "Eating, LDL oxidation, and coronary artery disease," www.ajcn.org/cgi/reprint/68/4/759.pdf

No authors listed, "Risks and Benefits of Estrogen Plus Progestin in Healthy Postmenopausal Women: Principal Results From the Women's Health Initiative Randomized Controlled Trial," *JAMA* 2002;288:321-333.

No authors listed, "Research update: Omega-3 EPA and DHA," *Nutritional Outlook*, 2003 Jan/Feb:80.

Nordoy A, et al., "n-3 polyunsaturated fatty acids and cardiovascular diseases," *Lipids* 2001;36 Suppl:S127-9.Moss, Ralph W, *Antioxidants Against Cancer*, Equinox Press, Gilroy, CA.

Nygård O, Nordrehaug JE, Refsum H, et al., "Plasma homocysteine and mortality in patients with coronary artery disease," *New England Journal of Medicine* 1997; 337: 230-6.

O

Olsen RB, et al., "Social networks and longevity. A 14 year follow-up study among elderly in Denmark," *Soc Sci Med* 1991;33(10):1189-95.

Ou P, Tritschler HJ, Wolff SP, "Thioctic (lipoic) acid: a therapeutic metal-chelating antioxidant?" *Biochem Pharmacol* 1995 Jun 29;50(1):123-6.

P

Palan PR, et al., "Plasma concentrations of coenzyme Q10 and tocopherols in cervical intraepithelial neoplasia and cervical cancer," *Eur J Cancer Prev* 2003 Aug;12(4):321-6.

Patrick L, "Mercury toxicity and antioxidants: Part 1: role of glutathione and alpha lipoic acid in the treatment of mercury toxicity," *Altern Med Rev* 2002 Dec;7(6):456-71.

Pauling, Linus, How To Live Longer and Feel Better, Avon Books, 1996.

Pauling, Linus, and Ewan Cameron, *Cancer and Vitamin C*, The Linus Pauling Institute of Science and Medicine, Menlo Park, CA:1979.

Paulmyer-Lacroix O, et al., "Glucocorticoids, 11 beta-hydroxysteroid dehydrogenase type 1, and visceral obesity," *Med Sci (Paris)* 2003 Apr;19(4):473-6.

Pert, Candace; *Molecules of Emotion*, 1997. Touchstone Books, New York, NY, USA, page 321.

Peterson JC, Spence JD, "Vitamins and progression of atherosclerosis in hyper-homocyst(e)inaemia," *Lancet* 1998 351: 263.

Pierpaoli, Walter, MD, PhD, William Regelson, MD, and Carol Colman, *The Melatonin Miracle*, Simon and Schuster, New York NY:1995.

Pollan, Michael, "The (Agri)Cultural Contradictions of Obesity," *NY Times Magazine*, October 12, 2003.

Portakal O, et al., "Coenzyme Q10 concentrations and antioxidant status in tissues of breast cancer patients," *Clin Biochem* 2000 Jun;33(4):279-84.

Pruthi S, Allison TG, Hensrud DD, "Vitamin E supplementation in the prevention of coronary heart disease," *Mayo Clin Proc* 2001 Nov;76(11):1131-6.

Pianin, Eric, "Toxins cited in farmed salmon: cancer risk is lower in wild fish, study reports," *Washington Post* 2004 Jan 9:A1

R

Ramos M, Wilmoth J, "Social relationships and depressive symptoms among older adults in southern Brazil," *J Gerontol B Psychol Sci Soc Sci* 2003 Jul;58(4):S253-61.

Reid RL, "Progestins in HRT: impact on endothelial and breast cancer," *J SOGC* 2000 Sep;22(9):677-81.

Reiter, Russell R, and Robinson, Jo; *Melatonin*, 1996. Bantam Books, New York, NY, USA.

Renaud S, Lanzmann-Petithory D, "Dietary fats and coronary heart disease pathogenesis," *Curr Atheroscler Rep* 2002 Nov;4(6):419-24.

Ridker PM, Morrow DA, "C-reactive protein, inflammation, and coronary risk," *Cardiol Clin* 2003 Aug;21(3):315-325.

Ridker PM, et al., "Homocysteine and risk of cardiovascular disease among postmenopausal women," *JAMA* 1999;281:1817-1821.

Rimm EB, et al., "Folate and Vitamin B6 from Eating and Supplements in Relation to Risk of Coronary Heart Disease among Women," *JAMA* 1998;279:359-364.

Rijnkels JM, et al., "Photoprotection by antioxidants against UVB-radiation-induced damage in pig skin organ culture," *Radiat Res* 2003 Feb;159(2):210-7.

Rimin EB, et al., "Vitamin E consumption and the risk of coronary heart disease in men," *NEJM* 1993;28:1450-6.

Rosano GM, et al., "Natural progesterone, but not medroxyprogesterone acetate, enhances the beneficial effect of estrogen on exercise-induced myocardial ischemia in postmenopausal women," *J Am Coll Cardiol* 2000 Dec;36(7):2154-9.

Rosmond R, "Stress induced disturbances of the HPA axis: a pathway to Type 2 diabetes?" *Med Sci Monit* 2003 Feb;9(2):RA35-9.

Roussow JE, et al., "Risks and benefits of estrogen and progestin in healthy postmenopausal women: principal results from the Women's Health Initiative randomized controlled trial," *JAMA* 2002 Jul 17;288(3):321-33.

Rubin, Rita, "Report is the latest case against HRT," *USA Today,* Tuesday, March 18, 2003:8D.

S

Saldeen TG, Mehta JL, "Dietary modulations in the prevention of coronary artery disease: a special emphasis on vitamins and fish oil," *Curr Opin Cardiol* 2002 Sep;17(5):559-67.

Sapolsky RM, *Why Zebras Don't Get Ulcers,* New York: Freeman and Company, 1994;37-58.

Sapolsky RM, Alberts SC, Altmann J, "Hypercortisolism associated with social subordinance or social isolation among wild baboons," *Arch Gen Psychiatry* 1997 Dec;54(12):1137-43.

Satta A, et al., "Effects of ubidecarenone in an exercise training program for patients with chronic obstructive pulmonary diseases," *Clin Ther* 1991 Nov-Dec;13(6):754-7.

Schiffmann, Erich, "The Line of Perfect Flow," *Yoga Journal,* January/February 1998, San Francisco, CA, USA.

Seeman TE, et al., "Social network ties and mortality among the elderly in the Alameda County Study," *Am J Epidemiol* 1987 Oct;126(4):714-23.

Seeman TE, et al., "Social relationships, social support, and patterns of cognitive aging in healthy, high-functioning older adults: MacArthur studies of successful aging," *Health Psychol* 2001 Jul;20(4):243-55.

Seeman TE, Berkman LF, "Structural characteristics of social networks and their relationship with social support in the elderly: who provides support," *Soc Sci Med* 1988;26(7):737-49.

Selley ML, "Increased concentrations of homocysteine and asymmetric dimethylarginine and decreased concentrations of nitric oxide in the plasma of patients with Alzheimer's disease," *Neurobiol Aging* 2003 Nov;24(7):903-7.

Shabsigh R, "Hypogonadism and erectile dysfunction: the role for testosterone therapy," *Int J Impot Res* 2003;15Suppl4:S9-S13.

Shah P, et al., "Lack of suppression of glucagon contributes to postprandial hyperglycemia in subjects with type 2 diabetes mellitus," *J Clin Endocrinol Metab* 2000 Nov;85(11):4053-9.

Shults CW, et al., "Effects of CoQ10 in early Parkinson's disease: slowing of the functional decline," *Arch Neurol* 2002 Oct;59(10):1541-50.

Shute WE, *Vitamin E Book*, Keats Publishing, New Canaan CT: 1978.

Simpson H, Savine R, Sonksen P, et al., "Growth hormone replacement therapy for adults: Into the new millennium," *Growth Horm IGF Res* 2002;12:1-33.

Singh RB, et al., "Randomized, double-blind placebo-controlled trial of coenzyme Q10 in patients with acute myocardial infarction," *Cardiovasc Drugs Ther* 1998 Sep;12(4):347-53.

Singh RB, et al., "Effect of hydrosoluble coenzyme Q10 on blood pressures and insulin resistance in hypertensive patients with coronary artery disease," *J Hum Hypertens* 1999 Mar;13(3):203-8.

Singh RB, et al., "Effect of coenzyme Q10 on risk of atherosclerosis in patients with recent myocardial infarction," *Mol Cell Biochem* 2003 Apr;246(1-2):75-82.

Skerrett PJ, Hennekens CH, "Consumption of fish and fish oils and decreased risk of stroke," *Prev Cardiol* 2003 Winter;6(1):38-41.

Smith KR, Zick CD, "Linked lives, dependent demise? Survival analysis of husbands and wives," *Demography* 1994 Feb;31(1):81-93.

Snowdon DA, et al., "Serum folate and the severity of atrophy of the neocortex in Alzheimer disease: findings from the Nun study," *American Journal of Clinical Nutrition* 2000 Apr;71(4):993-8.

Snyder PJ, et al., "Effect of testosterone therapy on body composition and muscle strength in men over 65 years old," *J Clin Endocrinol Metab* 1999 Aug;84(8):2647-53.

Snyder PJ, et al., "Effect of testosterone therapy on bone mineral density in men over 65 years old," *J Clin Endocrinol Metab* 1999;84(6):1966-72.

Stephens NG, et al., "Randomised controlled trial of vitamin E in patients with coronary disease: Cambridge Heart Antioxidant Study (CHAOS)," *Lancet* 1996;347:781-6.

Sternbach H, "Age-associated testosterone decline in men: clinical issues for psychiatry," *Am J Psychiatry* 2000 Feb;157(2):307-8.

Stipp, David, "The Secret Killer: Scientists believe they may have found a common link in diseases from cancer to Alzheimer's to heart disease. Hre's the story behind the search for that link," *Fortune,* Monday, October 13, 2003.

Sturm, Roland, "Increases in clinically severe obesity in the US, 1986-2000," *Arch Intern Med* 2003;163(18):2146-2148.

T

Tapiero H, et al., "I. Arginine," *Biomed Pharmacother* 2002 Nov;56(9):439-45.

Tenover JS, "Declining testicular function in aging men," *Int J Impot Res* 2003 Aug;15 Suppl 4:S3-8.

Tenover JS, "Prevalence and management of mild hypogonadism: introduction," *Int J Impot Res* 2003, Suupl 4, S1-S2.

Tenover JS, "Male hormone replacement therapy including 'andropause,'" *Endocrinol Metab Clin North Am* 1998 Dec;27(4):969-87.

Thies F, et al., "Association of omega-3 polyunsaturated fatty acids with stability of atherosclerotic plaques: a randomized, controlled trial," *Lancet* 2003 Feb 8;361(9356):477-85.

Thomas MJ, "The molecular basis of growth hormone action," *Growth Horm IGF Res* 8:3-11.

Thomas AM, "Growth hormone and cardiovascular disease: An area in rapid growth," *J Clin Endocrinol Metab* 2001;86:1871-1873

Tower RB, Kasl SV, Darefsky AS, "Types of marital closeness and mortality risk in older couples," *Psychosom Med* 2002 Jul-Aug;64(4):644-59.

Tucker JS, et al., "Marital history at midlife as a predictor of longevity: alternative explanations to the protective effect of marriage," *Health Psychol.* 1996 Mar;15(2):94-101.

U-V

Uno N, et al., "Neurotoxicity of glucocorticoids in the primate brain," *Horm Behav* 1994 Dec;28(4):336-48.

Urban RJ, et al., "Testosterone administration to elderly men increases skeletal muscle strength and protein synthesis," *Am J Physiol* 1995 Nov;269(5 Pt 1):E820-6.

Vance ML, Mauras N, "Growth hormone therapy in adults and children," *New Engl J Med* 1998;341:1206-1216.

VanGorp T, Neven P, "Endometrial safety of hormone replacement therapy: review of literature," *Maturitas* 2002 Jun 25;42(2):93-104.

Venkateswaran V, Fleshner NE, Klotz LH, "Synergistic effect of vitamin E and selenium in human prostate cancer cell lines," *Prostate Cancer Prostatic Diseases* 2004 Jan 27:Epub.

Verhoef P, et al., "Plasma total homocysteine, B vitamins, and risk of coronary atherosclerosis," *Arteriosclerosis, Thrombosis, and Vascular Biology,* 1997;17:989-995.

Visioli F, et al., "Lipoic acid and vitamin C potentiate nitric oxide synthesis in human aortic endothelial cells independently of cellular glutathione status," *Redox Rep* 2002;7(4):223-7.

Vittinghoff E, "Risk factors and secondary prevention in women with heart disease: the Heart and Estrogen/Progestin Replacement Study," *Ann Intern Med* 2003 Jan 21;138(2):81-9.

Voko Z, et al., "Dietary antioxidants and the risk of ischemic stroke: the Rotterdam study," *Neurology* 2003 Nov 11;61(9):1273-5.

von Kane IR, et al., "Effects of psychological stress and psychosomatic disorders on blood coagulation and fibrinolysis: a biobehavioral pathway to coronary artery disease?" *Psychosom Med* 2001 Jul-Aug;63(4):531-44.

W-Z

Walton KG, et al., "Stress reduction and preventing hypertension: preliminary support for a psychoneuroendocrine mechanism," *J Altern Complem Medicine* 1995;1(3):263-83.

Wiernsperger NF, "Oxidative stress: the special case of diabetes," *Biofactors* 2003;19(1-2):11-8.

Wilson AD, et al., "Primary sensory neuronal rescue with systemic acetyl-L-carnitine following peripheral axotomy. A dose-response analysis," *Cochrane Database Syst Rev.* 2003;(2):CD003158.

Wilkinson EG, et al., "Bioenergetics in clinical medicine. VI. adjunctive treatment of periodontal disease with coenzyme Q10," *Res Commun Chem Pathol Pharmacol* 1976 Aug;14(4):715-9.

Willman, David, "Stealth Merger: Drug Companies and Government Medical Research," December 7, 2003:A1.

Winslow R, "Heart Disease Hits the Preschool Set: New Research Shows Warning Signs Begin In Early Childhood," *Wall Street Journal* 2003 Tues March 18:D1.

Woo, Michelle M. M.; Tai, Chen-Jei; Kang, Sung Keun; Nathwani, Parimal S.; Pang, Shiu Fun; and Leung, Peter C. K.; "Direct Action of Melatonin in Human Granulosa-Luteal Cells," *The Journal of Clinical Endocrinology and Metabolism*, vol. 86 no. 10, October 2001, pages 4,789-4,797.

Writing Group for the Women's Health Initiative Investigators; "Risks and Benefits of Estrogen Plus Progestin in Healthy Postmenopausal Women," *The Journal of the American Medical Association*, vol. 288 no. 3, July 17, 2002, pages 321-333.

Wu D et al., "Age-associated increase in PGE2 synthesis and COX activity in murine macrophages is reversed by vitamin E," *Am J Physiol* 1998 Sep 27(3 Pt 1):C661-8.

Zandi PP, et al., "Reduced risk of Alzheimer disease in users of antioxidant supplements: the Cache County study," *Archives of Neurology* 2000; 61:82-8.

Zebrack JS, Anderson JL, "The role of inflammation and infection in the pathogenesis and evolution of coronary artery disease," *Curr Cardiol Rep* 2002 Jul;4(4):278-88.

Zozaya JL, "Nutritional factors in high blood pressure," *J Hum Hypertens* 2000 Apr;14 Suppl 1:S100-4.

INDEX

A

AA (arachidonic acid), 82-83, 86
AAMI (age-associated memory impairment), 119
adrenal glands, 123
adult-onset diabetes. *See* type 2 diabetes
affirmations, 31
Age Optimization, 22-23
aging, 18, 60
  biology of, 57
  body changes, 58
  theories of, 59
    caloric restriction theory, 63
    cross-linkage theory, 64
    disposable soma theory, 59
    genetic control theory, 62
    Hayflick limit theory, 63
    immunity theories, 64
    neuroendocrine theory, 61
    rate of living theory, 63
    telomerase theory, 62
    waste accumulation theory, 61
    wear and tear theory, 60
ALA (alpha linolenic acid), 88
ALA (alpha lipoic acid), 115-17
ALC (Acetyl-L-Carnitine), 115, 118-20
  in animal studies, 120
  benefits of, 119
alpha lipoic acid, 66, 107-8, 115-18
Ames, Bruce, 116
anastrozole, 129
andropause, 125
anger, 44, 48-51, 53
Anger: Wisdom for Cooling the Flames (Hanh), 102
Anti-Inflammation Zone, The (Sears), 83
antioxidants, 66, 108
antioxidant system, 66
  reduction, 66
apoptosis, 101
Arimidex, 129
aromatization, 128-29
atherosclerotic plaques, 149
Atkins, Robert, 80
Avodart, 128
awareness, 15, 18-19, 24-25, 35, 44, 80
awareness exercises, 26

B

beliefs, 27-29, 31
Berman, Jennifer, 179
beta-amyloid, 127
beta-endorphin, 97
bio-identical hormone therapy. *See* hormone replacement therapy
Blackburn, Elizabeth, 62
BMI (body mass index), 58, 75-76
BPH (benign prostatic hypertrophy), 128-29
breast cancer, 133, 142
  indole-3-carbinol, 142
  Premarin, 142

C

carbohydrate addiction, 97
carbohydrates, 75, 94-95, 97
   complex, 95-97
   refined, 68, 75, 92, 95, 97
cardiovascular disease, 69, 71, 92
Castaneda, Carlos, 18
CFS (chronic fatigue syndrome), 148, 154
Chinese medicine, traditional, 71
cholesterol, 85, 91-92
   HDL, 91-92
   LDL, 91-92
chromium picolinate, 107
Cisplatin, 119
coenzyme Q10, 115
collagen, 64, 68
conscious eating, 102
consciousness, 18
CoQ10 (coenzyme Q10), 66, 92, 115-16
cortisol, 48, 63, 147, 150-51, 153, 155
   benefits and risks, 151
cosmic intelligence, 36
C-reactive protein, 75, 83, 93
C-RP (C-reactive protein), 75
Cushing's disease, 153

D

dehydroepiandrosterone, 148
DHA (docosahexaenoic acid), 89, 120
DHEA (dehydroepiandrosterone), 147-50
   risks, 149
DHT (dihydrotestosterone), 128
diabetes, 68-71, 84, 96, 118, 158

diet, 20
   low-glycemic, 98, 154
dihydrotestosterone, 128
docosahexaenoic acid, 120

E

eating
   sacredness, 35
ED (erectile dysfunction), 126, 149, 182
eicosanoids, 80-87, 89-90, 93
   balancing, 87-89
   function, 87
eicosapentaenoic acid, 83, 120
Einstein, Albert, 56
emotions, 33
endorphins, 168, 177
endothelium, 142
EPA (eicosapentaenoic acid), 83, 120
Epel, Elissa, 62
erectile dysfunction, 96, 139, 149, 181-83
   drugs, 182
   elastic bands, 182
   emotions, 183
   penile prostheses, 182
   vacuum devices, 182
   vitamin B6 supplements, 183
estradiol, 100, 127, 129, 136, 141
estriol, 136
estrogen, 122, 124, 126, 132, 138
   flavors, 136
estrogen dominance, 137
exercise, 163, 174
   aerobic exercise, 169
   a few tips, 165
   intensity, 169-70
   interval training, 170

Kegels, 167, 183
  spiritual benefits, 166
  strength training, 169, 172
  yoga, 172
exercise literacy, 167

F

failure, 31-32
fats, 85
  belly, 75, 82-83
  partly saturated, 85
  saturated, 85, 89-90, 92
  trans fats, 86, 90-91
  unsaturated, 76, 85
fatty acids, 65, 85-86
  omega-3, 86-88, 90, 115
  omega-6, 86-88
fear, 31, 47-49
  neurotic, 29
feelings, 32-34
  Jung's theory, 34
fiber, 68, 94-95
fibrin, 69
fibromyalgia, 114, 154
food literacy, 19-21, 73-74
foods, 35, 45, 72-73
  fast food, 72
  impact on the body and mind, 80
  junk food, 72
forgiveness, 49, 51
free radicals, 65-66
fructose, 94, 98

G

galactose, 94
genes, 62, 83, 101

GHRH (growth hormone-releasing hormone), 159
GI (glycemic index), 97-99
gingivitis, 93
glucagon, 80, 82, 93, 96, 151
glucose, 65, 94-95, 151
glucose-6-phosphate dehydrogenase, 149
glutathione, 66, 117
glycation, 65, 67-68
Glycemic Food Index Guide, 5, 195
glycerol, 85
goiter, 155
growth hormone deficiency, 157
guidelines
  optimal eating, 97, 99
  optimal eating, low calorie, 99
  optimal eating, low-glycemic, anti-inflammatory, 97
gum care, 93
  periodontal disease, 93, 116

H

habits, 79
Hanh, Thich Nhat, 102, 180
  Anger: Wisdom for Cooling the Flames, 102
health literacy, 15, 18-20
heart attack, 69
heart rate, calculating, 170-71
hemoglobin, 168
herbs
  anti-inflammatory, 101
  curcumin, 101
  ginger, 101
  for prostate enlargement, 129

HGH (HUMAN GROWTH HORMONE), 124, 147, 153, 157-59
  enhancing production, 159
  replacement, 158
homocysteine, 110
hormone replacement, 124-25
hormone replacement therapy, 13, 125, 132-34, 136, 189
  estrogen, 136, 139, 143
    breast cancer, 142
  melatonin, 160-61
  for men, 122
  progesterone, 137-39
  testosterone, 130-31
  for women
    long-term benefits, 141
    short-term benefits, 140
hormones, 84, 123-24, 147
  ideal range, 191-92
  supplements, 123
  testing, 124
HRT (hormone replacement therapy), 133-34, 142, 144
Human growth hormone, 157-59
hydrogenation, 90
hydroxytyrosol, 90
hyperglycemia, 68, 70
hyperhomocysteinemia, 110
hyperthyroidism, 155-56
hypothalamus, 123
hypothyroidism, 155-57

I

I3C (indole-3-carbinol), 100, 142
immune system, 64
indole-3-carbinol, 100, 142
infertility, 137

inflammation, 65-68, 82-84
  chronic, 67, 82-83, 101
  fever, 66-67
insulin, 80, 82, 95
insulin levels, chronic spiking of, 95
insulin resistance, 68, 70, 96, 118, 158

J

JABS (judgment, anger, blame, and shame), 53
Jung, Carl
  on feeling, 32
  on projection, 41

L

Lee, John, 137
Lesnikov, Vladimir, 159
Levothroid, 157
levothyroxine, 157
Levoxyl, 157
libido, 149
lipoprotein(a), 91
love, 46-49
lycopene, 101, 115
  carotenoid, 101

M

Maffetone, Philip, 170
male menopause. *See* andropause
meditation, 173-74
melatonin, 147, 159-62
Melatonin (Reiter and Robinson), 162
Melatonin Miracle, The (Pierpaoli), 162
mercury contamination, 88, 113

metals, heavy, 88, 117
mindfulness, 12, 174
minerals, 111-12
   calcium, 112-13
   magnesium, 113-14
   selenium, 114
mistakes, 32, 38
mitochondria, 65
Molecules of Emotion (Pert), 17, 36-37

N

N-acetyl-cysteine, 118
National Social Life, Health and Aging Project (NSHAP), 139
neuropathy, 117
nitric oxide, 118
norepinephrine, 48
nutritional supplements, 104-5, 107
   cons, 106
   need for, 105
NVC (nonviolent communication), 53
   judgment, anger, blame, and shame, 53

O

obesity, 68, 77-78
   physical conditions, 78
   war on, 23
obesity epidemic, 76
oils
   flax oil, 88
   hydrogenated, 90
   monounsaturated, 89-90
   olive oil, 85, 89-90, 96, 101
   polyunsaturated, 90
omega-3 fats, 120

omega-6 fats, 88
osteoporosis, 112, 153
oxidation, 65, 68, 84

P

Paclitaxel, 119
pain, 38
Pert, Candace, 17, 36-37
   Molecules of Emotion, 17, 36-37
pharmaceuticals, 14
Pierpaoli, Walter
   Melatonin Miracle, The, 162
pineal glands, 160
pituitary gland, 124, 158
plaque, 69-70, 111
polycystic ovary syndrome, 137
Premarin, 133-35, 142
Prempro, 133
progesterone, 122, 124, 126, 132, 138
progestins, 132-35, 142
   synthetic, 134
projection, 41-43, 55
Prometrium, 138, 144
Propecia, 128
Proscar, 128
prostaglandins, 182
PSA (prostate-specific antigen), 128
psychoneuroimmunology, 36

R

RealAge: Are You as Young as You Can Be? (Roizen), 70
Regelson, William, 159
Reiter, Russell J., 161-62
relationships
   with food, 43, 45
   healthy, 51

interpersonal, 40, 45
  right relationship, 42, 44, 46
  wrong relationship, 44
  with your body, 44
  with yourself, 45
respect, 54
Robinson, Jo, 162
Roizen, Michael, 70
  RealAge: Are You as Young as You Can Be?, 70
Rubner, Max, 63

S

sacrifice, 21-22
safrole, 161
Sapolsky, Robert, 153
Schiffman, Erich, 172
sciatica, 118
Sears, Barry, 80, 83
  Anti-Inflammation Zone, The, 83
  zone plan, 81, 189
self-talk, 26, 30-31
Semmelweis, Ignaz, 81
serotonin, 97
sex hormones, 122
sexual activity, benefits, 177
sexual anxiety, 178
sexual difficulties
  men, 181
    erectile dysfunction, 181
  women, 183
    libido, 183
    vaginal dryness, 183
Sexual Healing, 5, 176
sexuality, 139, 177, 179-80, 184
  communication, 178
  feelings, 180
  spending time together, 181
  touch, 184
SHBG (sex hormone binding globulin), 126, 139-40
simple sugars, 68, 80, 88, 94, 96
  disaccharides, 94
  monosaccharides, 94
  oligosaccharides, 94
  polysaccharides, 94
SIP (silent inflammation profile), 83
starches. *See* carbohydrates, 94
statin drugs, 91-92, 115, 134
steroids, 126
stress, 49, 64, 152
  fight-or-flight response, 47-48, 151, 153, 169
  signs, 152
  ways to alleviate, 154
stroke, occlusive, 70
Sturm, Roland, 76
Synthroid, 157

T

TCM (traditional Chinese medicine), 71
telomeres, 62-63
temptation, 77
testosterone, 122, 124-32, 139-40
  aromatization, 129-30
  bio-identical, 130
  bound, 126
  brain and, 127
  free, 124, 126, 128, 140
  health and bone health, 127
  male vigor, 125-26
  in men, 122, 125
  prostate and, 128
  in women, 122, 132, 140, 142
tests

blood tests, risk for heart disease, 192
C-reactive protein test, 83
salivary hormone tests, 143, 150
standard, 191
thyroid-stimulating hormone test, 157
vertical auto profile, 92
thoughts, 35-36
thrombosis, 87, 134
thyroid hormone, 147, 155
 synthetic, 157
Thyroid Hormone Testing, 157
thyroid imbalance, 155-57
time, 18
 chronos time, 18, 55
 kayros time, 18, 55
triglycerides, 85, 92
TSH (thyroid stimulating hormone) test, 157
2-OHE, 100
type 2 diabetes, 68-70

V

vaginal dryness, 133-34, 138, 183
vanity, 55
VAP (vertical auto profile), 92
vitamins, 108
 B vitamins, 110-11
 vitamin C, 110
 vitamin E, 109

W

What Your Doctor May Not Tell You About Breast Cancer (Lee and Hopkins), 137
What Your Doctor May Not Tell You About Menopause (Lee and Hopkins), 137
What Your Doctor May Not Tell You About Premenopause (Lee and Hopkins), 137